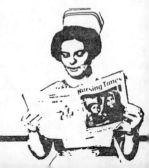

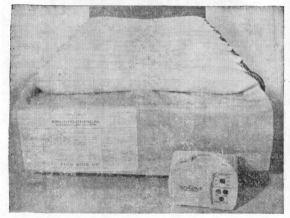

Qualified Nurses for the Royal Navy

The nurses of QARNNS care for naval personnel and their families. Their work can take them to any part of the world in which there is a naval base. There are direct entry schemes for qualified nurses.

Nursing Officers

S.R.N.'s with at least two years' post-registration experience. Preference will be given to those with an extra qualification.

Naval Nurses

Qualified S.E.N.'s under the age of 28.
Pay is good and there are six weeks annual leave.
In addition, the Royal Navy has first-class sports and social facilities.

For further information please write to: Matron-in-Chief, Queen Alexandra's Royal Naval Nursing Service, Empress State Building, London SW6 1IR.

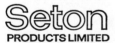

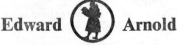

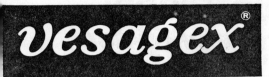

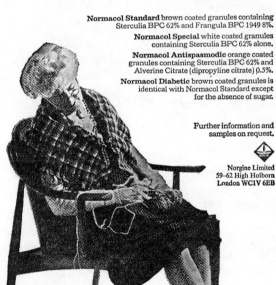

BAILLIÈRE'S POCKET BOOK OF

Ward Information

BY

Marjorie Houghton,† OBE

Formerly Education Officer, the General
Nursing Council for England and Wales;
and Sister Tutor, University College Hospital,
London

REVISED BY

L. Ann Jee, SRN, Part 1 CMB, RNT

Examiner to the General Nursing Council
for England and Wales; Member of the
Area Nursing Training Committee, Manchester
Region; and Nurse Tutor, Park Hospital,
Davyhulme, Manchester

Twelfth Edition

Baillière Tindall · London

© 1971 Baillière, Tindall & Cassell Ltd.
7 & 8 Henrietta Street London WC2

Twelfth edition 1971

Reprinted 1973

Reprinted 1976

Reprinted 1977

This book, originally written by Dr. H. L. Heimann and Dora Wilson as *The Nurses' Pharmacopoeia*, was first published in 1933. Their sixth edition appeared in 1949. As the *Pocket Book of Ward Information* it was revised for the seventh edition in 1953 by Marjorie Houghton, who saw the book through to the eleventh edition in 1965. This was reprinted in 1968.

ISBN 0 7020 0351 4

Published in the USA by
The Williams & Wilkins Company
Baltimore 2, Maryland

*Printed in Great Britain by Cox & Wyman Ltd.
London, Fakenham and Reading*

Preface

This book contains many facts, figures, definitions and descriptions of basic procedures which the nurse will find useful for study and for quick reference when on duty in the ward. It is a tribute to the work and scholarship of the late Marjorie Houghton, author of many editions, who condensed so much useful information into so small a space. Times change, however, and new material has had to be introduced, but in preparing this new edition I have tried to keep to the spirit and purpose of the book.

At the beginning the nurse will find a section on emergencies and related procedures, which offers guidance on the treatment of cardiac arrest, asphyxia, pulmonary embolism, haemorrhage, and attempted suicide. With this I have included a description of cardiac monitoring, which is increasingly undertaken in the ward and not only in intensive care units. For this same reason, I have provided some notes on dialysis. I have taken account of new drugs, new diagnostic procedures, the change-over to the metric system, and modern vaccination and immunization practice. Throughout I have kept in mind my nursing colleagues working in remote areas overseas who may not always have advanced equipment available, and I have tried to balance the conflicting demands of teaching and reference needs, and the limitations of space imposed by ever rising costs.

In the preparation of this edition I am indebted to many of my nursing and medical colleagues in Park Hospital, in particular to Miss Janet Boey, Clinical Teacher at Park Hospital, who advised me on current ward practices, Miss T. Clarke, Group Pharmacist, West Manchester Hospital Group, and Mrs D. Swinnerton, Clinical Teacher of the Christie Hospital and Holt Radium Institute, for her advice on radiotherapy.

November 1970   L. ANN JEE

Contents

1 Emergencies and Related Procedures

The nurse may sometimes find herself in a situation in which an important decision must be taken quickly. Each hospital lays down its own rules about the responsibilities a nurse may take upon herself, even in an emergency: each nurse should therefore familiarize herself with the rules laid down by her own hospital. Unless it is absolutely unavoidable, due to extreme urgency, she must seek advice from a doctor or a senior member of the nursing staff, and if this is impossible she should ask another member of the nursing staff to witness her actions. In any case, she must always inform a senior nurse of any decision she has made on her own initiative, at the earliest opportunity.

Whatever the emergency, the ability to think clearly and act calmly is a valuable asset: shouting and confusion not only frighten patients but may upset other members of the ward team.

In cases of collapse of a patient the usual routine is:

(1) To check the patient's airway.
(2) To summon help (according to the instructions laid down by the hospital).
(3) To see that the Resuscitation Trolley (or box) is at the bedside and open.
(4) To treat for shock. (If giving oxygen, make sure the right mask is used; see p. 17.)

At the first appropriate moment, the nurse must reassure a conscious patient; she must also remember that many unconscious patients can still hear what is being said.

Cardiac Arrest

This is the sudden unexpected and total failure of the heart to pump blood around the body. Common causes are: post operative shock, electrocution, coronary thrombosis, or an overdose of a drug. The brain is the most sensitive organ to lack of oxygen and will die if circulation is not restored within 3 to 4 minutes at normal temperature. The signs of cardiac arrest are:

(1) Unconsciousness; gasping or absent breathing.
(2) Absent pulses.
(3) Greyish cyanosis with pallor developing later.
(4) Dilated pupils in most cases.
(5) Twitching and a brief major fit in some cases.

Cardiac Resuscitation

The patient should be placed on his back on a hard surface, the airway cleared and dentures removed; and the legs may be raised to assist venous return. A sharp blow to the sternum may be effective in restarting the heart beat. If not, place one hand flat, with the heel of the other hand over it, both pressing with elbows straight over the lower end of the sternum. A rhythmic swinging forward of the shoulders depresses the sternum by about 1½″. This squeezes the heart against the vertebral column. The movement is repeated about 60 times a minute. Mouth to mouth respiration is started simultaneously; one lung inflation should alternate with five chest compressions. If a nurse is working alone the ratio of fifteen to three is recommended. In infants one or

AN OUTLINE OF ACTION FOR SOME COMMON EMERGENCIES

Emergency	Danger	Action
Asphyxia (see also p. 6)	Oxygen deprivation leading to cardiac arrest and brain damage	1. Clear airway 2. Give artificial respiration 3. Treat for shock
Cardiac arrest (see also p. 2)	Brain damage unless circulation restored within 3–4 minutes at normal temperature	1. Clear airway 2. Give artificial respiration simultaneously with cardiac massage 3. Treat for shock
Pulmonary embolism (see also p. 7)	Fatal collapse	1. Reassure patient 2. Assist patient into comfortable position for breathing and support 3. Give oxygen 4. Treat for shock
Sudden haemorrhage (see also p. 9)	Excessive blood loss	1. Where possible apply pressure directly or indirectly. Raise injured limb 2. Prepare for intravenous therapy and/or possible return to theatre 3. Give oxygen if patient pale or breathless 4. Give reassurance and prepare for possible injection of morphine 5. Treat for shock

Note: In all cases follow the routine procedure where applicable (see p. 1) both thumbs are applied over the middle of the sternum and light compression (about 12 mm or $\frac{1}{2}''$) is at the rate of 100 to 120 per minute.

The Cardiac Monitor (or Oscilloscope)

This is a machine by which a continuous visual recording or electrocardiogram (ECG) is made of the heart's rhythm. The machines vary from a portable one with a very small screen to a much larger one incorporating such refinements as alarm systems and printed recordings of the ECG. They may be used for patients following cardiac arrest, coronary thrombosis or cardiac surgery.

The nurse is not expected to master the intricacies of the machine on first contact for this needs special training and experience. If an opportunity arises, she should familiarize herself with the essential controls and study the tracing of the patient on the machine so that she can at least recognize a deviation from the normal rhythm without necessarily diagnosing the cause or knowing the treatment. She should avoid conveying any apprehension she may feel to the patient and his relatives.

The monitor is an aid to nursing and the nurse is still required to make very careful and accurate observations on her patient. The machine cannot record changes such as colour, temperature, character of respiration or distress in the patient which are observations of value to the doctor. Major arrhythmias are often preceded by minor ones and the observant nurse, by reporting such a deviation, can give valuable help to the doctor who can then prevent or anticipate complications.

The equipment consists basically of the following parts:

Two main cables: one leads to the mains plug; the second one contains about 3 to 5 leads.

The leads: each carry terminals at their tips.

The terminals: these are attached to the electrodes which in turn are attached to the patient's limbs or chest.

The electrodes: for the limbs these are usually small flat metal discs which are stuck to the patient's skin with special jelly and secured by a rubber strap. The terminals are attached to them. Those for the chest vary in size and shape according to the manufacturer and may be disposable. The area of skin under the electrode should be shaved if necessary and very thoroughly cleaned each day before the electrodes are applied. If the electrodes are not thoroughly cleaned, there may be interference with the electric circuit. The doctor decides the position of the electrodes but in an emergency it is helpful if the nurse can affix them quickly. Some are labelled and others have coloured leads as a guide to their position on the patient's body.

If a flat line appears on the screen and it is obvious that the patient has not suffered a cardiac arrest, the connections, leads and electrodes must all be carefully checked for disturbance. Other electrical apparatus placed too near the monitor, or undue muscular movement of the patient can interfere with the tracing on the monitor. When the straps securing the limb electrodes are applied too tightly, they are uncomfortable, but if too loose they may alter the tracing.

The patient may require a battery powered unit called a pacemaker which discharges electrical impulses to his heart via a catheter electrode passed through a vein in the arm or neck to the right ventricle. The size of the pacing impulse may also be recorded on the monitor.

Care is needed to prevent infection tracking along the catheter route and this is prone to displacement. Failure of the battery results in an emergency as the stimulation causing the heart to beat regularly will have ceased.

The nurse who is able to project herself into the needs of the patient rather than being over-concerned with the machine will gain the patient's confidence and so influence his chances of recovery.

Asphyxia

When breathing stops through interference with the normal levels of oxygen and carbon dioxide in the body, this may be caused by obstruction of the airway, paralysis of the respiratory muscles due to drugs, gases or disease, collapse of lung tissue, or replacement of air content by fluid, e.g. in drowning or with inhaled vomit. Artificial ventilation is required. Many methods are available, some suitable for emergency situations and short periods only, whilst others are designed for longer periods (see p. 19).

Artificial Airways

In most hospitals, a Brook airway is readily available. This is similar to the airway used in anaesthetized patients but it contains a seal to cover the patient's mouth and a one-way valve is incorporated. This is preferable to the direct mouth-to-mouth method, particularly if the patient has a chest infection. Many hospitals provide a simple type of self-inflating bag, for example an Ambu bag which can be attached to the Brook airway. This can be used until medical help is available. Other types of equipment are constructed, so that oxygen can be delivered to the patient via a face mask.

Mouth-to-Mouth and Mouth-to-Nose Methods

The patient must be lying on his back with the nurse standing at his side, or kneeling if he is on the floor. The mouth and throat should quickly be cleared of any foreign material, particularly dentures. With one hand on the forehead and the other under the neck, the head is tilted back as far as possible, this position being maintained throughout. The nurse's lips form a wide seal round the patient's mouth and the cheek is pressed firmly against the nose to seal it or the nostrils can be pinched. Air is then blown into the mouth until the patient's chest rises. He is then left to breathe out through his mouth and nose. The first ten breaths are given as rapidly as possible and the rate should then be between 12 and 15 times a minute.

An alternative method is to seal the mouth and breathe into the nose. It is said that there is less likelihood of blowing air into the stomach by this route.

In infants and babies the lips should cover both mouth and nose, and the resuscitator must breathe gently and *not* too deeply if she is to avoid damage to the delicate lung tissue.

Pulmonary Embolism

This occurs when a blood clot, air bubble or fat embolus becomes detached from its anchor, usually in the pelvic or calf veins and travels to the lungs. The severity depends upon the size of the clot dislodged, and may vary from a temporary chest pain and breathlessness and cyanosis to a sudden fatal collapse. It may follow surgery, particularly that undertaken in the pelvic area, or be associated with congestive heart failure.

The patient is usually very frightened and needs reassurance. He should be assisted into a position where respiration is most comfortable for him, and be well supported. Oxygen must be administered quickly but the nurse must bear in mind that patients with a history of respiratory difficulty such as that associated with congestive heart failure and cor pulmonale will need a venti mask.

Sudden Haemorrhage

This may follow operation as a result of a ligature slipping from a main vessel but it may also occur as a massive haematemesis or haemoptysis. Medical aid must be sought immediately as delay in returning a patient to theatre or replacing blood loss in time, could be fatal to the patient. Until the doctor arrives carry out the usual First Aid measures, apply pressure and raise limbs as appropriate to reduce blood flow. Sometimes a nurse may justifiably apply a tourniquet, but she must be prompt in informing the doctor of her action. Treat for shock and reassure the patient.

Treatment for Shock

The four emergencies above are usually accompanied by severe shock, which needs to be treated as soon as breathing and heart beat have been restored.

Shock may be defined simply as a decrease in the effective circulating blood volume or acute hypotension. The treatment will be of the cause, but a nurse can help by ensuring that the patient has a clear airway, is lying in most cases and is covered but not overheated. In severe shock, the patient's veins may collapse quickly, making the administration of intravenous fluid difficult for the doctor. It is therefore helpful and time saving if the nurse has the intravenous equipment ready when the doctor arrives.

Blood pressure is lowered in cases of shock but it may also be lowered by the action of drugs given specifically by the anaesthetist during surgery to assist the surgeon. Where a low blood pressure persists, venous return is assisted by raising the foot of the bed. Blood flow is more important than blood pressure in these particular cases but the nurse's observations are important and a systolic blood pressure recording below 60 mm Hg must be reported to the doctor immediately.

Attempted Suicide

A patient may attempt to commit suicide in many ways. The observant nurse may well sense the patient's intention and so anticipate the action. Clear thinking, a calm but firm manner and a quiet sympathetic voice are of more value than stern or censorious behaviour towards a patient on the verge of precipitate action. A nurse who is alone should never attempt to restrain a very agitated or violent patient, except from making a physical attack on patients around him. Planned restraint with several assistants and a syringe containing, for example, a prescribed dose of haloperidol (Serenace) or promazine hydrochloride (Sparine) may be necessary. Attempted suicide is also a psychological emergency and a nurse who takes an informed interest in her patients' problems may be able to give psychological support when the first emergency is ended.

Accidents in the Ward

It is customary in most hospitals for an Accident Form to be completed at the earliest opportunity if, for example, a patient falls out of bed. In spite of protestations on the patient's part that he is not hurt, the nurse

must report the accident immediately and seek medical
aid.

Notes on Administrative Procedures

Nurses are sometimes asked to witness Wills or to give
information to the Press. In many hospitals nurses are
expressly forbidden to do either, and they should know
the rules of their own hospital.

The age of consent for the administration of an anaesthetic, 16 years, is an acceptable age for certain procedures, but many surgeons prefer the consent also of
husband, wife or parent for operations such as therapeutic abortion, sterilization, hysterectomy, amputation
and certain other procedures. The decision not to apply
cardiac resuscitation is primarily that of the doctor in
charge of the case. Where any doubt exists, the nurse
must carry out the procedure until medical opinion has
been sought.

It is wise for a nurse to have a witness with her when
dealing with the possessions of an unconscious patient.
In the event of an orthodox Jewish patient dying sud-
denly, a Gentile nurse should not touch the body until
the wishes of the relatives have been sought. When a
patient of the Roman Catholic faith dies unexpectedly,
his priest should be informed within the hour so that
he may administer Holy Unction. Relatives of a patient
who has died unexpectedly should always be asked if
they would like to see a minister of religion: his particular training equips him to give consolation in times
of distress.

2. Treatment of Poisoning

The most common poisonings today are due to hypnotics, tranquillizers, antidepressants, salicylates and carbon monoxide gas.

All containers or utensils which may have contained the poison and all material ejected by the patient should be carefully preserved for examination. In many cases of self-poisoning, a mixture of drugs is taken.

The first aim of treatment is to dilute and remove the poison if at all possible. If this cannot be done, as is obviously the case if the poison has been injected and is already absorbed into the blood stream, then the aim must be to neutralize the effects of the poison or to render the poison inert. At the same time every effort should be made to combat the effects of the poison which may be endangering life; for example, if respiratory failure is present it must be treated without delay.

Respiratory Failure

This is liable to occur in poisoning due to barbiturates and other hypnotic drugs, in carbon monoxide and prussic acid poisoning. Maintenance of a clear airway is the first essential, the patient being nursed in the usual post-operative position. Some doctors prefer the head to be lower than the feet particularly where there is a risk of aspiration of vomit. Depending on the degree of unconsciousness, a cuffed endotracheal tube may be inserted. If the patient is cyanosed oxygen should be given. If there is any risk of carbon dioxide retention, a venturi mask will be used. Artificial respiration may be necessary and if this is required for more than about

11

30 minutes, a mechanical respirator will be needed (see p. 19). Occasionally it may be necessary to give 2 ml of nikethamide (Coramine) I.M. to stimulate respiration temporarily whilst other methods are being prepared. Tracheostomy is seldom necessary unless endotracheal intubation is needed for longer than 48 hours.

If elevation of the lower limbs is ineffective in raising the systolic blood pressure above 90 mm Hg, other treatment may be instituted. It is thought that various mechanisms operate in these cases to produce a reduction in the venous return to the heart and one of the best ways of restoring blood pressure here is to give a vasoconstrictor drug such as metaraminol (Aramine) I.M. 5 mg at 20-minute intervals. Intravenous fluids are not always desirable.

Assessment of the Patient for Treatment

The patient is assessed on the degree of unconsciousness and the presence or absence of other medical complications such as shock or respiratory failure. Some patients who have become habituated to a drug are able to tolerate a much higher blood level of the drug before becoming unconscious or suffering the ill effects than those who are not habituated, for example epileptics taking phenobarbitone. Patients suffering from acute salicylate poisoning rarely become unconscious. In adults therefore, even drowsiness must be regarded as a dangerous sign. Children are more likely to become drowsy or unconscious. If there is any doubt about the amount of the drug ingested, biochemical assessment must be undertaken without delay.

The successful outcome of treatment in roughly 95% of cases of poisoning is that of intensive nursing care of the unconscious patient. The remaining 5% of cases will require more specialized techniques of treatment such as forced diuresis or dialysis.

Treatment

Dilution of the poison. In the majority of cases water is the most readily available fluid for the dilution of a swallowed poison. The victim should be encouraged to drink as much as possible, 4 tumblers or more. Milk is also a suitable diluent particularly in the case of corrosive or irritant poisons since it has a demulcent action, protecting the mucous membrane and hindering the absorption of the poison.

Removal of the poison. Within 4 hours of ingestion and in any cases of salicylate poisoning, very thorough stomach lavage is the most effective method and this may be carried out with plain warm water (38° C). Where corrosive poisons have been swallowed, this may be undertaken in selective cases with caution; a doctor's advice should be sought. In cases of petrol or paraffin poisoning 30 ml of liquid paraffin should be swallowed prior to the lavage and the patient is then encouraged to swallow milk to which approximately 5 g of sodium bicarbonate has been added. Castor oil, if it is easily available, can be added to the lavage water in cases of phenol poisoning. This dissolves the phenol, thereby delaying absorption.

Where possible in the case of the unconscious patient, intubation with a cuffed endotracheal tube should precede the lavage. The procedure is then easier and the position not so important. Where this is not possible, the patient is best positioned face down with his head lower than his body to avoid the risk of the fluid being aspirated into the air passages. A wide bore gastric tube should be slightly lubricated and passed through the

mouth. About 300 ml water is passed through a funnel
before being siphoned back.

Emetics are not as efficient as gastric lavage but may
be the quickest remedy available. The immediate use of
emetics is contra-indicated in corrosive poisoning. A
useful emetic can be made from 1 tablespoonful of
common salt or mustard dissolved in a tumbler of warm
water.

Poisons Information Service

In Britain the Poisons Information Service gives advice
and information on the treatment of specific poisons to
general practitioners and hospitals. This covers substances used in the home, agriculture, industry and
medicine. A comparable service is also available in
Europe, Australia and the U.S.A.

Telephone numbers of Poisons Information Service

Belfast	0232 30503
Cardiff	0222 33101
Dublin	Eire, Dublin 45588
Edinburgh	031-229 2477
Leeds	0532 32799
London	01 407 7600
Manchester	061 740 2254
*Newcastle upon Tyne	0632 25131

---

*This service has been temporarily suspended. In the meantime in-
formation is available from the Pharmacy Department at the same
number (Monday to Friday, 9 a.m. to 5 p.m.; Saturday, 9 a.m. to 1 p.m.).

3. Oxygen Therapy

The administration of oxygen is needed in conditions where the normal supply of oxygen to the tissue cells cannot be maintained. This may be due to respiratory difficulties, circulatory failure, or to the inability of the red blood cells to combine with oxygen, as happens in the case of carbon monoxide poisoning. Examples of common conditions in which oxygen is either essential or beneficial are pneumonia, collapse of the lung (atelectasis), pulmonary emphysema, cardiac and thoracic surgical operations, congestive cardiac failure and any condition producing severe shock.

Fire Precautions

Although oxygen itself does not burn, any material which burns in atmospheric air will burn much more easily if the concentration of oxygen in the air is increased. Therefore certain precautions should be strictly observed.

Patients and visitors should be warned against smoking or lighting matches in the vicinity. No electrical bells, lights or heating pads should be allowed inside an oxygen tent. Children should not be given mechanical toys. Hair should not be vigorously combed. Patients should not wear nylon nightdresses. The patient must not be rubbed with oil or spirit whilst the tent is being operated. Should this procedure be necessary the oxygen flow must be discontinued during the time that the treatment is being carried out.

Oil or grease of any description must not be used on

the oxygen cylinder or fittings. The nozzle of the cylinder must be cleaned before attaching the regulator.

Oxygen Cylinders and Fittings

For purposes of identification oxygen and other medical gas cylinders are painted in distinctive colours and the name and/or symbol of the gas is stencilled on the cylinder. The table on p. 17 gives the standard colours as issued by the British Standards Institute.

Oxygen is compressed into cylinders of different sizes at 132 atmospheres, which is an equivalent of approximately 1,940 lb per square inch. This pressure must be reduced prior to administration to a patient. Wherever possible an automatic oxygen regulator should be employed for this purpose, but when not available a fine adjustment valve may be used with care. A litre gauge or flowmeter is necessary in order that the prescribed rate of flow may be maintained. These gauges may be of the dial or the bobbin type. In the latter a bobbin inside a graduated glass tube rises as the oxygen passes through and the height of the bobbin against the scale shows the amount of oxygen being delivered. The flowmeter is usually incorporated in the cylinder fittings with the pressure gauge and regulator.

Before attaching the regulator to the cylinder the cylinder valve should be opened slightly, so that any grit or dust that may have accumulated may be blown out. The regulator is then fitted into the head of the cylinder by inserting the threaded end into the valve opening and tightening it by means of the winged nut. The litre gauge should be turned off and the cylinder opened slowly until the cylinder contents gauge shows 'full', the cylinder is then opened completely by giving the key one more turn. The cylinder is then ready for use.

In many wards the oxygen supply is delivered by a pipeline to each bed, but every ward should possess at least one oxygen outfit ready for immediate use. The cylinder, in a wheeled stand with the fittings and the apparatus for delivering the oxygen to the patient, should be regarded as emergency apparatus which must always be kept in working order. An empty cylinder should be clearly marked 'EMPTY' when removed and it should be replaced at once by a full cylinder.

Identification Colours for Medical Gas Cylinders

		Colour	
Gas	*Symbol*	*Top*	*Body*
Oxygen	O_2	White	Black
Nitrous oxide	N_2O	Blue	Blue
Cyclopropane	C_2H_6	Orange	Orange
Carbon dioxide	CO_2	Grey	Grey
Ethylene	C_2H_2	Violet	Violet
Helium	He	Brown	Brown
Nitrogen	N_2	Black	Grey
Oxygen and carbon dioxide mixture	O_2+CO_2	White and Grey	Black
Oxygen and helium mixture	O_2+He	White and Brown	Black
Air	—	White and Black	Grey

These colours are laid down by the British Standards Institution.

Disposable Masks

Different types of plastic disposable apparatus are now available for the administration of oxygen.

Oxygen is also used in conjunction with aerosol sprays containing bronchial dilator drugs, antibiotics or substances which help in the easier expectoration of sputum. These too are inhaled for a limited period through a face mask.

Face masks. These are light in weight and cover the nose and mouth; some are rigid whilst others are soft and flexible. For maximum efficiency, they must fit the patient's face closely but comfortably. Perspiration tends to accumulate on the patient's face and if this causes distress, the mask can be lifted occasionally and the face wiped quickly. The rate of flow, ordered by the doctor, varies between 4 and 8 litres per minute.

Venti and Venturi masks. These masks, which have a rigid base with a flexible face area, are used for patients with chronic lung disease, which in some cases is also associated with congestive heart failure. The respiratory centre in these patients has become conditioned to a higher concentration of carbon dioxide due to decreased oxygen intake. These masks are so constructed that the amount of oxygen the patient receives does not exceed 28%, or in some cases 35%. This amount raises the oxygen in the blood sufficiently for the patient to benefit. Higher concentrations such as those achieved by use of the oxygen tent or other face masks could be fatal to these patients.

Nasal tubes. Two nasal catheters are attached to a Y-shaped tube, the stem of the Y being connected to the oxygen supply. The catheters are passed about 2½ cm (approximately 1″) along the floor of the nose. They can be passed into the nasopharynx, but this method often produces discomfort for the patient although it increases the concentration of oxygen. If necessary, the nostrils may first be cleaned with sodium bicarbonate solution and cocaine ointment applied to relieve discomfort.

A similar apparatus is made in disposable soft plastic material.

It is necessary to moisten the oxygen when the nasal route is used, by passing the gas through a humidifier.

This method is less efficient than administration by the face mask, as the concentration of oxygen is lower and breathless patients tend to breathe through the mouth. The advantages are that the mouth is left free for drinking or cleaning and it is also useful for those patients who need to expectorate.

Mechanical Ventilators

Where prolonged ventilation is necessary, there are now many types of mechanical ventilator in use. The majority work on the principle of intermittent positive pressure; an endotracheal tube is used for short periods or a tracheostomy tube for longer periods.

These machines are constructed to pump air, oxygen or other gases rhythmically to and from the patient's lungs. According to the various needs of the patient, the machine can be regulated to control the volume at inspiration and expiration; some, known as 'breathing assisters', are triggered by the patient's own respiration and take up his rhythm of breathing. The rate and pressure of breathing can also be controlled and the air humidified with the aid of mechanical devices. These machines at first sight may appear very complicated to the unpractised nurse, but given the opportunity to observe the machine in action together with instructions regarding the function of the appropriate valves, she can soon become familiar with the aspects important to the successful nursing of the patient. In the event of a power failure, the nurse must know how to work the machine manually.

The following observations are usually made:

(1) Chest movement. If the chest wall is not rising in time with the respirator's action, tubing should be checked to see that it has not become disconnected. If the patient breathes spontaneously out of phase with the ventilator, the nurse should notify the doctor who may consider discontinuing the use of the ventilator or may give a muscle paralysing agent to allow the ventilator to control respiration entirely.

(2) Colour. If cyanosis occurs the doctor must be informed.

(3) Blood pressure, pulse and respiration rates are noted.

(4) Volume of air given at each inspiration is noted.

(5) Expired volume of air per minute is noted, together with the positive and negative pressures of the machine.

(6) Pupil reaction. The nurse should remember that tubocurarine does not affect pupil reaction.

(7) If there is a rising positive pressure obstruction may be present, or the patient may be attempting to breathe spontaneously. Tubing should be checked for kinking. Water which collects in the loops of the tubing should be emptied. Suction should be applied to the trachea. If no cause is found, the doctor must be notified.

(8) If there is a falling positive pressure, all tubing must be checked for air leaks, particularly at con-

nections and at the cuff of the endotracheal or tracheostomy tube.

(9) The temperature within the humidifier and the level of sterile distilled water must be checked and maintained at normal.

(10) The observations related to the general nursing care of a patient will of course be made, and particular attention should be given to the pressure areas and to the mouth.

Other respirators, originally known as 'iron lungs' work on the same principle as physiological respiration· They are also known as Negative-Positive pressure respirators. A large pump rhythmically withdraws air from the cabinet in which the patient is enclosed and then allows it to return. In this way air is alternately drawn into the patient's lungs and then expelled as in normal respiration. Although these models have been much improved in recent years, it is thought that the negative-pressure inside the cabinet tends to draw blood away from the heart. Nursing treatments are also difficult to carry out as the patient must be completely enclosed from the neck downwards inside the cabinet. If bulbar paralysis develops, the patient is in danger. The saliva which collects in his naso pharynx due to his inability to swallow, can be sucked into his lungs as the pressure changes from negative to positive and this could ultimately asphyxiate the patient.

Oxygen Tents

The tent method of administering oxygen is used for children more than for adults. There are several different types in use. Essentially the tent consists of a canopy of transparent plastic material mounted on a wheeled frame

with metal stretchers to support the head of the canopy:
there are openings in the canopy through which the
nurse's arms can reach the patient for any necessary
attention. Cooling of the air inside the tent is effected
by passing the air through an ice box or through a
refrigeration unit, and in some types of tents the carbon
dioxide is removed by passing the air through a container of soda-lime.

A full cylinder of oxygen ready for use, as described
on p. 16 and, where necessary, a supply of ice should be
obtained before erecting the tent. A wall thermometer to
record the temperature inside the tent, which should
usually be maintained at 18° to 21° C, will also be required.

If the tent has an ice cabinet the ice is broken into
pieces about the size of a man's fist and the ice container
filled to capacity. About 3 feet of rubber tubing is then
connected to the water outlet of the ice cabinet and a pail
is placed under the rubber drainpipe. The ice cabinet is
raised so that it will be clear of the ground when the
canopy is fitted; the lid of the cabinet must be securely
fastened otherwise there will be a leak of oxygen. A
water seal is provided in the cabinet to prevent oxygen
leaking through the drainpipe. The head of the canopy
must be securely attached to the openings provided on
the ice cabinet, this is done by means of rubber inserts
or rubber corrugated tubing.

The back of the canopy has a nozzle marked 'oxygen.
inlet' to which the rubber tubing from the cylinder
regulator is attached. This should be done and the flow
adjusted to five litres a minute before the canopy is
placed over the patient. The temperature control should
be set to 'cold'. Two persons are needed to fit the
canopy over the patient's bed. The height of the tent and

cabinet must be adjusted so that the head of the canopy will be about 15 cm (6″) above the patient's head. The skirt of the canopy is lifted and spread out so that it covers the bed and can be tucked in all round. The openings of the canopy in most tents have zip fasteners, otherwise they are sealed by rolling them up and securing the flaps with bulldog clips.

As the tent is set up the oxygen flow should be turned on until the needle of the litre gauge registers 'flush' and this full flow is then allowed to continue for about 5 minutes, after which time the flow is reduced to the dosage ordered, which may be from 4 to 8 litres per minute. All patients, and children in particular, should be provided with a hand bell. Many feel a sense of claustrophobia or isolation, so that where possible, continuous or very frequent observation should be employed.

Some tents have an electric motor incorporated which forces the oxygen to circulate, allows greater control of the temperature and improves the ventilation inside the tent.

When an oxygen tent is dismantled after use the canopy should be mopped with a disinfectant solution and then washed with soap and water.

When high humidity conditions are required 'Humidaire' type oxygen tents are very satisfactory.

Suction

Most wards are provided with suction machines. Small hand-operated bellows may be used in an emergency or whilst moving a patient but they are not as effective as a machine. The ideal position for the patient is with the head slightly extended. This prevents the catheter entering the oesophagus instead of the trachea, when the

swallowing reflex is still present. The patient's head is
turned to one side and then to the other to introduce the
catheter into each bronchus: this avoids the natural
tendency of the catheter to enter the right bronchus. The
suction machine is turned on to the required pressure
and the sterile catheter connected to a Y connection on
the tubing leading from the machine. It should be
handled with forceps or a gloved hand. It is then introduced into the nasal passages and passed gently on-
wards until it reaches the excess secretions. At this point,
the nurse covers the open end of the Y connection on
the tubing and withdraws the catheter gently so that
suction is applied as the catheter is withdrawn. This prevents the mucosa adhering to the end. Failure to handle
the catheter gently may result in bruising or even haemorrhage within the trachea. If the patient coughs during
the procedure, the sputum expectorated at that time
must be aspirated. The nurse should observe and report
on the character of the sputum aspirated. Suction must
not be prolonged because this causes discomfort to the
patient. If suction by this method is not satisfactory,
bronchoscopy may be required.

If the suction apparatus is incorporated into an intermittent positive pressure machine, the suction must be
switched off immediately after use as it affects the running of the respirator.

Disposable catheters are discarded after use, non-
disposable catheters should be cleared by flushing
through with sodium bicarbonate solution before the
machine is turned off. They may then be soaked in a
solution of sodium bicarbonate before being re-
sterilized. The same procedure applies when a tracheostomy tube is in position, the suction catheter being
passed via the tracheostomy tube.

Oxygen for a Patient with a Tracheostomy Tube

When a patient has had a tracheostomy performed it is obvious that he cannot benefit by oxygen given by a face mask or by nasal tubes.

A Perspex collar which fits round the patient's neck over the tracheostomy tube is available (Oxygenaire). An opening in the front of the collar with a 'pear-drop' cover allows suction to be carried out with the collar in position. Perforations at the side of the collar permit the escape of expired air and also allow the patient to continue to breathe atmospheric air should the oxygen supply accidentally fail.

If the oxygen collar is not available then oxygen must be given through a catheter passed into the opening of the tracheostomy tube.

Under certain circumstances the nursing staff will be instructed to deflate the cuff on the tracheostomy tube at regular intervals. The procedure should be as follows:

The patient's mouth should be cleansed and the machine then disconnected. The suction catheter is introduced into the trachea and the cuff is deflated immediately afterwards. Any secretions that may have trickled past the cuff are then aspirated, after which the machine is re-connected. The cuff is reinflated after five minutes with just enough air to prevent leakage around it. Over-inflation can cause damage to the trachea.

The nurse may be asked to introduce a measured amount of a specified fluid down the tracheostomy tube hourly or at specified times. After introducing the fluid, the plug is replaced and the patient is allowed three breaths. By manipulating the Y tube of the catheter, suction is then applied during withdrawal. It should be possible to introduce the fluid and to suck out thoroughly in about thirty seconds. It is important that the patient should not be left off the machine for longer periods than this.

Hyperbaric Oxygen

Special chambers or tanks are needed for the administration of oxygen which is raised to 2 or 3 atmospheres, so that the blood may become super saturated with a high tension of dissolved oxygen. This may be used for such cases as carbon monoxide poisoning, gas gangrene, or myocardial infarction.

4. Fluid and Electrolyte Balance

In health the amount of fluid in the body and its composition remains remarkably constant, in spite of variations in intake, but in almost every case of serious illness
or extensive surgical operation the balance can be grave-
ly disturbed and may need restoring urgently. For this
reason one of the nurse's most valuable contributions to
the treatment of the patient is an accurate 24-hour
record of all fluid going into the patient and all fluid
output, including the volume, the route and the type of
fluid.

The Water Content of the Body

The total quantity of water in the adult body amounts
to approximately 70% of the total body-weight. Two-
thirds of this water is inside the cells, intracellular
fluid, one-third is outside the cells, the extracellular
fluid; most of the latter is contained in the blood plasma
and the interstitial fluid, lymph, which bathes the tissue
cells. An adult weighing 70 kilograms (11 stone) contains in his body about 50 litres of fluid weighing 50 kg;
of this total about 34 litres are intracellular fluid and
16 litres extracellular. Approximately 5% of the total
body-weight is accounted for by the water content of the
blood, i.e. 3·5 litres.

Substances in Solution—Electrolytes

Many substances are contained in solution in the body
fluids; some of these, such as glucose, provide food for
the cells, others, such as urea, are the waste products of

the cell metabolism and must be removed in solution in the water surrounding each cell. The interstitial fluid must be able to effect an exchange with the blood plasma as well as with the intracellular fluid in order to transfer to the cell those substances that it needs and to clear waste products from the cell into the blood.

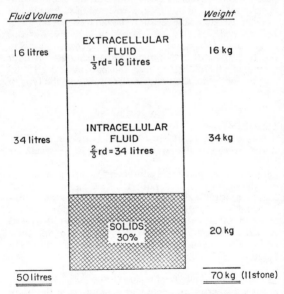

APPROXIMATE PROPORTIONS OF FLUIDS
AND SOLIDS IN THE ADULT BODY

Intracellular and extracellular fluids both contain salts in solution, the presence of which in the correct concentration is responsible for the interchange of material through the semipermeable (or differential permeable) membrane which forms the cell boundary and maintains the normal tension within the cell. These all-important salts form electrolytes (i.e. in solution they

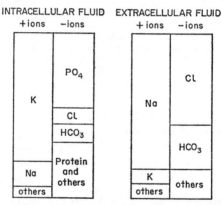

INTRACELLULAR FLUID   EXTRACELLULAR FLUID

COMPARISON OF ELECTROLYTES IN THE INTRACELLULAR
AND THE EXTRACELLULAR FLUID

dissociate into electrically charged particles, or ions). Some ions carry a positive charge and are known as cations, others are negatively charged and are called anions. The chief cations in the body fluids are sodium (Na), potassium (K), calcium (Ca), and magnesium (Mg). The chief anions are chloride (Cl), bicarbonate (HCO_3)

and phosphate (PO_4). The electrolytes in the extracellular fluid are mainly sodium and chloride, while the intracellular fluid contains mainly potassium and phosphate and a little chloride.

The concentration of electrolytes in the body fluids can be measured and is usually expressed in units known as milliequivalents per litre (mEq/l). The measurement of the concentration of electrolytes is expressed in mEq/l because chemicals react by equivalent and not by absolute weight. The word equivalent means literally 'equal valency' and relates the valency of any particular chemical to that of hydrogen. The equivalent weight of a substance is the atomic weight divided by its valency and is expressed in grammes; the milliequivalent is therefore expressed in milligrams. To give one example of the chemical use of these calculations, the normal value for potassium in the blood plasma is 4·5 mEq/l. In some conditions, including acute renal failure, it is essential to check the blood potassium level; if it rises to 7 mEq/l or higher there is grave danger of cardiac arrest.

Normal Values of Blood Electrolytes

Constituent	Value/100 ml of plasma	mEq/litre
Sodium	310–340 mg	136–145
Potassium	14–20 mg	3·5–5·0
Chloride (as Cl)	350–375 mg	100–106
Bicarbonate (HCO_3)	57–75 Vol %	24–28
Calcium	9–11 mg	4·5–5·5
Phosphorus	3–4·5 mg	—

Acid-Base Balance—pH Scale

The pH formula gives the concentration of hydrogen ions in solution; acid solutions have a higher concentration of these ions than alkaline solutions. The pH scale runs from 0 to 14, the higher the hydrogen ion concentration the lower the reading; 7 represents neutrality—if a solution gives a reading below this figure it is acid, above 7 the solution is alkaline.

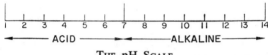

THE pH SCALE

The maintenance of the normal reaction of both the extracellular and the intracellular fluids in terms of acidity or alkalinity is another factor which governs the health of the cells. The reaction of the extracellular fluid is normally slightly alkaline and this is expressed as a pH value of about 7·4, a range of 7·35 to 7·45 on this scale being within normal limits. Intracellular fluid is slightly acid but its reaction is not known precisely.

The reaction of both extracellular and intracellular fluids remains very constant in health. Urine, however, has a variable reaction and although usually slightly acid, it can vary between 4·7 and 8. This is because one of the main functions of the kidneys is to maintain the normal reaction of the body fluids and to excrete any excess of either acid or base. The terms 'acidosis' and 'alkalosis' are frequently used and denote in the first case that the blood contains more acid than normal and in the second case it contains an excess of base.

Daily Requirements for Water and Electrolytes

An adult excretes about 1 litre of urine in 24 hours and also loses about 1 litre through the lungs in expired air, through the skin as perspiration and in the water content of faeces. He therefore needs to take in at least 2 litres of fluid daily to make good this loss. No harm results from an excessive intake of fluid in health as the kidneys are well able to dispose of unwanted fluid, a fact with which everyone is familiar. If there is an excessive loss of water, as for example by heavy sweating, this will normally be made good almost immediately; the individual feels thirsty and drinks freely.

The minimal requirement of sodium chloride is not known, but the average intake of 5 g (80 mEq.) represents an enormous excess over the minimum. We are therefore not likely to be deficient in health since we all take common salt with our food. Potassium and other salts are also present in sufficient amounts in a normal diet. In illness both water and salt often need to be given intravenously. Acute potassium losses are usually replaced intravenously, chronic losses orally in the form of potassium chloride, or potassium bicarbonate.

In many conditions diminished intake is accompanied by excessive loss of water and electrolytes, for example by vomiting, diarrhoea, gastric aspiration, polyuria, plasma or blood loss. Treatment must therefore be planned to cover this loss as well as lowered intake, and allowances must be made for losses which have occurred before treatment started. Accurate intake and output records and repeated blood electrolyte estimations are essential features of successful replacement therapy.

Treatment of Fluid and Electrolyte Disturbance

In practice these disturbances are usually multiple, affecting the water content, electrolytes and acid-base balance simultaneously. For clarity of description, however, it is convenient to consider the most important factors and their appropriate treatment separately.

1. Water

(a) *Water depletion*. This may be due to excessive loss, diminished intake or a combination of both; loss of fluid may not be obvious, as for example in intestinal obstruction when large quantities can collect in the distended intestine in addition to fluid lost by vomiting. Depletion due to lowered intake is particularly liable to occur in comatose, or semi-comatose, patients. Lack of water is characterized by thirst, dry mouth and tongue and decreased urinary output. In severe cases, where it is usually accompanied by sodium deficiency, the patient has a pale, anxious face with sunken eyes: the extremities are cold and may be cyanosed: the skin loses its elasticity and in infants the fontanelle is depressed. The pulse rate is then usually increased and the blood pressure low. Water depletion can be corrected by giving fluid by mouth or intragastric tube, if the patient's condition permits, or by the intravenous administration of a 5 % glucose solution in water. In cases with accompanying electrolyte loss, however, the type of fluid to be given will be determined after estimation of the blood electrolytes.

(b) *Excess of water*. Excess of water, or 'water intoxication', usually results from the administration of large quantities of fluids to patients whose urinary output is inadequate. The effects of water intoxication are due to increased tension within the cells and the clinical manifestations are mental confusion, convulsions and coma. Muscle cramps may also occur. Chronic intoxication produces oedema of the lungs and systemic oedema. The condition can be produced by the rectal administration of tap water or glucose solutions. Water intoxication can be prevented if an accurate intake and output chart is kept and the fluid given is restricted, in the case of an adult, to a maximum of 1 litre plus the volume of the urinary output over the previous 24 hours. If the symptoms are severe the condition may be treated by vigorous water restriction, and occasionally by the intravenous administration of hypertonic (5%) sodium chloride solution.

2. Sodium

(a) *Sodium depletion.* Depletion may occur as a result of prolonged vomiting, gastric or intestinal aspiration or drainage, diarrhoea, excessive loss of salt in the urine as in the polyuria of diabetic ketosis, in Addison's disease and in some cases of chronic nephritis. It may also occur as a result of ion-exchange resins; e.g. in heart disease. It is characterized by loss of elasticity of the skin, low intraocular pressure and, when severe, by low blood pressure, circulatory failure, apathy, confusion and shock. Sodium loss can be made good by the administration of salt by mouth or intravenous infusion of normal (isotonic) saline solution.

(b) *Sodium excess.* Excess may be present in cardiac failure and in the nephrotic syndrome; it may be produced by the administration of large doses of cortisone or intravenous infusion of saline given rapidly or in excessive amounts. The effect of sodium excess is to cause oedema, which is most dangerous when it affects the lungs. Treatment is related to the cause.

3. Potassium

(a) *Potassium deficiency* (hypokalaemia). Lack of

potassium may be due to a low intake, persistent vomiting, gastric aspiration, Cushing's syndrome, diarrhoea, chronic renal disease, diabetic ketosis, excessive administration of cortisone, or occasionally to an adrenal tumour secreting aldosterone. The chief manifestations of potassium lack are muscular weakness, intestinal paralysis and myocardial failure. The deficiency may be made good by the administration of potassium by mouth as potassium chloride or potassium citrate. 15 ml of Mixture of Potassium Citrate (N.F.) contains 3 g of potassium (28 mEq.). Potassium can also be given intravenously as 0·2 or 0·3% solution of potassium chloride, provided that the urinary output is adequate and that the rate of administration does not exceed 1 litre in 24 hours.

(b) *Potassium excess* (hyperkalaemia). Potassium excess occurs in cases of anuria from any cause and in Addison's disease of the adrenal cortex. Its effect is to produce listlessness, mental confusion, numbness and tingling of the extremities. As the serum potassium level rises, there is grave danger of cardiac arrest, therefore in the above-mentioned conditions it is necessary to avoid giving potassium in any form. High serum potassium levels can be lowered by the administration of potassium-binding ion-exchange resin, sodium polystyrene sulphonate (Resonium-A) 7·4 g 4-hourly by mouth or Ryle's tube. The resin may also be given rectally to a vomiting patient in an emulsion of 30 g resin, 100 ml of 2% methyl cellulose and 100 ml water.

4. Bicarbonate

Changes in the bicarbonate (HCO_3) content of the plasma reflect disturbances in the acid-base balance of the body fluids.

(a) *Acidosis*. In this condition there is a tendency for the pH of the blood to fall. This may be due to the formation of acids (ketones) as in diabetic ketosis, the administration of acid-forming substances, such as salicylates, or decreased excretion of acid metabolites in renal failure. It may arise in hypothermia, when there is tissue anoxia and on recovery from cardiac arrest. Acidosis may also result from excessive loss of sodium and potassium as, for example, in cases of diarrhoea. In chronic respiratory disease, such as chronic bronchitis and emphysema, acidosis can occur from retention of carbon dioxide. Non-respiratory acidosis causes hyper-ventilation with deep sighing respirations, the 'acidotic breathing' seen in diabetic coma and uraemia, and leads to mental confusion and coma. Treatment consists of the appropriate therapy for the underlying condition, e.g. the administration of insulin in diabetic coma, and in chronic renal failure giving sodium bicarbonate, or sodium citrate, by mouth or normal (isotonic) saline solution intravenously. Alternative solutions for intravenous therapy are molar lactate or saline lactate solution, with or without potassium according to the needs of the individual case.

(b) *Alkalosis*. In this condition there is a tendency for the blood to become more alkaline than normal. Alkalosis may be due to excessive and prolonged administration of alkalis or to loss of hydrochloric acid from persistent vomiting or gastric aspiration. The amount of bicarbonate in the blood plasma increases and the clinical signs are anorexia, mental confusion, slow, shallow breathing and sometimes tetany; long-standing alkalosis may produce renal failure. The treatment is that of the precipitating cause. This condition is also treated with intravenous normal saline solution; if renal function is normal the kidneys will in this case retain the chloride and excrete the sodium. Potassium deficiency usually complicates alkalosis and this needs to be corrected simultaneously with sodium potassium chloride.

5. Intravenous Therapy, Blood Transfusion and Dialysis

Intravenous Infusion of Electrolyte Solutions

Replacement of large amounts of fluid lost from the body or the correction of serious electrolyte imbalance is most rapidly and accurately dealt with by the introduction of a suitable solution directly into the venous circulation. The solutions are individually prescribed and carefully checked during treatment by frequent blood examinations. Nutrients may also be given by the intravenous route (see p. 40). In all cases the rate of flow prescribed must be carefully maintained and an accurate record of the fluid given by this and by any other route and the patient's fluid output must be kept.

Central Venous Pressure

In some cases of severe shock due to sudden decreased blood volume, a change in the flow of blood returning to the heart is reflected by a fall in the venous pressure before it shows in a falling systolic pressure. By a means similar to that for cardiac catheterization (see p. 105) an indwelling catheter is passed into the (R) side of the heart, or if this is not possible, into the external jugular vein. The catheter is connected to a manometer, which is incorporated into the infusion apparatus. This provides a means of continuous assessment for fluid and electrolyte replacement.

For examples of intravenous solutions see p. 39.

Solutions used to provide Water and Electrolytes

Normal (isotonic)
  saline 0·9%
$\frac{1}{2}$ Normal saline
$\frac{1}{5}$ Normal saline
Hypertonic saline 5·85%
Bicarbonate solution
  8·4%
Glucose 5%
Glucose in $\frac{1}{5}$
  normal saline
Hartmann's solution

$\frac{1}{6}$ molar sodium
  lactate
Normal (isotonic)
  sodium lactate
Saline-lactate solution
  (for diabetic coma)
Potassium chloride
  in 2·5% glucose
Darrow's solution
Normal (isotonic)
  sodium bicarbonate

The same apparatus as that used for blood and plasma transfusions is suitable (see pp. 44 and 45) and the instruments required for cutting down on a vein may be required. Where the treatment is to be continued for several days a fine polythene tube which can be passed through a needle into the superficial vein and thence into a deep vein is usually preferred to a metal cannula, as there is then less likelihood of irritation of the vein wall and clot formation.

Blood, Plasma and Plasma Substitutes

Plasma, reconstituted.
Blood collected in sodium citrate solution.
  Fresh.
  After 10 days.
Dextran 6% in 5% glucose.
Dextran 10% in 5% glucose.
Dextran 6% in normal (isotonic) saline.

Proprietary Intravenous Solutions and their uses

Aminosol 10%   Essential amino acids and
                              mineral salts

Aminosol-Glucose   given as supplements
                              or nutritional additives in

Aminosol-Fructose   deficiency states.
  Ethanol

Fructose 20%

Vamin

Intralipid   A sterile fat emulsion
                              for intravenous use for
                              patients unable to
                              ingest adequate food orally.

Dextraven   Restoration of blood
                              volume.

Macrodex 6% in Normal Saline
  (Dextran 6% in Normal
  Saline)

Macrodex 6% in Dextrose   Plasma volume
  (Dextran 6% in 5%   expanders. Not
  Dextrose)   causing rouleaux

Rheomacradex 10% in Saline   or difficult blood
  (Dextran 10% in Normal Saline)   grouping.

Rheomacradex 10% in Dextrose
  (Dextran 10% in 5% Dextrose)

Mannitol   Osmotic diuretic not crossing the
                              cell membrane. In the kidney tubule
                              Mannitol leads to the elimination
                              of a certain amount of water bound
                              to it, causing osmotic diuresis.

Sorbitol   Hydrates a patient by intravenous
                              route also supplying a quantity of
                              carbohydrate Calories.

Proprietary foods taken by mouth are discussed on p. 119.

Blood and Plasma Transfusion

The usual indications for transfusion of blood or plasma are severe haemorrhage, burns and shock. Transfusion with whole blood or with concentrated red cells is also often required in the treatment of anaemia. The standard transfusion fluids provided by the Blood Transfusion Services of the United Kingdom are:

(1) Whole blood.
(2) Concentrated suspension of red blood cells.
(3) Dried plasma or serum, with sterile pyrogen-free fluid for reconstitution.

There are also a number of plasma substitutes, obtainable from commercial firms, which are widely used, for example a polysaccharide, Dextran.

Blood Groups

Transfusion of blood from one person to another is fraught with great risks unless it can be proved that the blood of the donor is compatible with the blood of the recipient. Every individual has substances in his blood which react against 'foreign' proteins, including, in some cases, the proteins in the blood cells of another human being. The effect of these antibody substances is to cause agglutination, or clumping, of the red blood cells. Sometimes, however, the individual will produce no antibodies in response to foreign red cells entering his blood stream and in this case the blood of the donor is said to be compatible with that of the recipient; in other words both these individuals belong to the same blood group. Human blood is, therefore, classified according to the type of red cell present and the most important classifications of these substances are known as the

ABO and the Rhesus (Rh) systems. Both donor and recipient must belong to the same ABO and Rh group. As a further check, since sub-groups may also be present, and because people acquire agglutinating bodies in addition to the 'natural' antibodies, it is also necessary to carry out direct tests matching the recipient's blood against the blood to be donated.

ABO system. Human blood falls into one of four ABO categories, A, B, AB or O. Groups AB and B are comparatively rare amongst European populations, most of whom belong either to the A or the O group.

Group A. This group has A antigens in the red cells and anti-B antibodies in the plasma.

Group B. This group has B antigens in the red cells and anti-A antibodies in the plasma.

Group AB. This group has both A and B antigens in the red cells but the plasma contains no anti-A or B antibodies.

Group O. This group has no A or B antigens in the red cells but has both anti-A and anti-B antibodies in the plasma.

Group A therefore cannot receive blood from Group B as the A group contains anti-B antibodies.

Group B similarly cannot receive from Group A.

Group AB has no anti-A or B antibodies and therefore, at least theoretically, can receive blood from all other groups.

Group O has both anti-A and anti-B antibodies and can therefore receive only Group O blood, but as Group O contains neither A nor B antibodies this group can give to all other ABO groups as the red cells of O group will not be agglutinated by the recipient's plasma.

Group O is sometimes referred to as the 'universal donor group' and may in cases of extreme emergency be given to a patient without awaiting the results of full cross-matching tests. In practice this is rarely done.

Rhesus group system. The Rhesus, or Rh group, was given this name as it was found that the same system of antibodies was present in the blood of the rhesus monkey. In this system the most important factor is labelled 'D'; the majority of Europeans have this D substance in their blood and are therefore described as Rh positive. About 15 % of the population, however, do not have the Rh factor and are said to be Rh negative; transfusion of Rh positive blood to a Rh negative individual can be dangerous, since the Rh negative blood will produce antibodies to destroy the transfused cells. The effect of a first transfusion may be slight, but the individual is liable to become sensitive to the D factor and further transfusions with Rh positive blood may produce a serious reaction. A similar reaction can take place in the blood of the fetus in cases where the mother's blood is Rh negative but that of the fetus is Rh positive. The maternal blood then produces antibodies which enter the fetal circulation via the placenta and destroy the fetal red blood cells. The fetus may die or, if surviving to term, the infant may be born with a severe type of haemolytic jaundice. Since sensitivity to the D factor takes some time to develop it is unusual for this reaction to occur in a first pregnancy. If a Rh negative girl or woman of child-bearing age is transfused with Rh positive blood this can also be the cause of a haemolytic reaction should the woman become pregnant with a Rh positive fetus, as her blood will in the meantime have produced Rh antibodies.

The bottles containing whole blood supplied by the Blood Transfusion Services are labelled to show the ABO and Rh groups, the date of collection of the blood from the donor and the date after which the blood is unfit for transfusion. Each bottle of stored whole blood contains 120 ml of an anticoagulant solution. Stocks for hospital blood banks and sterilized, disposable, giving sets are supplied from regional centres of the Blood Transfusion Services. Mobile units from these centres also arrange donor sessions, at a hospital or other convenient place, where blood is collected to maintain the stocks held at the regional centre.

Requirements for Transfusion

Container with the blood or other fluid as prescribed.

Recipient set—a sterilized 'disposable' nylon and polythene set which is used once and then discarded.

A small sterile pack containing towels and swabs.

Skin cleansing lotion.

Sphygmomanometer or a
    tourniquet to distend the superficial veins.

Adhesive strapping and scissors.

A polythene or similar sheet for protection of the
    bedclothes.

Instruments for cutting down on a Vein and tying in a Cannula

Scalpel or knife handle and blade.

One pair toothed fine dissecting forceps.

One pair non-toothed fine dissecting forceps.

One pair fine pointed scissors.

Two fine artery forceps.

Aneurysm needle.

Thread, size 60, or catgut, size 00.

Two curved skin needles and sutures.
Intravenous cannula or fine polythene tubing with an adaptor.
Hypodermic syringe, needle and local anaesthetic.
These instruments are usually supplied from a theatre or 'C.S.S.D.'

Clear instructions on the setting up of the apparatus are issued on the back of each container and these must be followed carefully. The tubing clamp is adjusted to give the required rate of flow. The intravenous needle or fine polythene tubing should be kept in position with adhesive strapping and the patient's arm or leg supported in a comfortable position on a protected pillow. In the case of infants, young children, or very restless patients it may be found necessary to splint the limb. The strapping or bandage used to fix the splint must be taken over bony prominences in order to avoid the risk of obstructing the venous circulation. The veins of the scalp may be used in infants instead of the veins in the arm or leg.

The use of a fine polythene cannula prevents immobility of the limb and the chance of the needle slipping out or piercing the vein wall.

Management of transfusions. In all cases where a blood transfusion is likely to be needed 5 ml of the patient's blood is obtained and sent to the laboratory for grouping and direct cross-matching tests with the sample of the blood to be transfused. Any error in the labelling of this specimen or the accompanying laboratory form could lead to incompatible blood being given.

The correct blood for the individual patient is then labelled with his full name, bed number, case notes number and ward, and the statement that the blood is

compatible is signed. The particulars on the label should
be checked when the bottle or bottles are removed
from the bank to the ward in order to ensure that
the right blood is given to the right patient. Almost
every case of incompatible transfusion is the result of
an administrative error, e.g. incorrect labelling, or
failure to check the label carefully, particularly when
there are two patients in the same ward with the same
name.

Stored blood must be kept at a temperature between
4° and 6° C (39° to 43° F) in a thermostatically controlled refrigerator. It should never be cooled below 4°C
or heated in any way. Bottles containing blood must
always be carefully handled to avoid shaking the contents, but it is permissible to mix the blood very gently
if the cells have settled to the bottom.

Whole blood may be used up to 21 days after withdrawal from the donor, provided that it is properly
stored. Red cell suspensions, which are prepared by
siphoning off the plasma from one or more bottles of
whole blood and pooling the red cells, must be used
within 24 hours of preparation.

Rate of flow of blood. Forty drops per minute is the
usual rate prescribed for a slow transfusion. Rapid
transfusion may be needed to replace a severe and
sudden loss of blood and in such cases one or more
bottles of blood may be given as rapidly as the blood
will flow into the vein. In extreme urgency intra-arterial
transfusion has been given, but is now little used.

Rate of flow of other fluids. The doctor may order the
infusion to be run through in a given number of hours.
Thus if 1 ml contains approximately 15 drops, the rate
at which a bottle containing 540 ml will run (allowing

for several ml which will remain behind) would work out as follows:

1 bottle in 4 hours — approx. 30 drops per minute
1 bottle in 6 hours — approx. 20 drops per minute
1 bottle in 8 hours — approx. 15 drops per minute

Changing bottles. The full bottle must be obtained from the bank and checked before the bottle in use is empty. The fresh bottle and a clamp forceps may be placed at the bedside. When the blood level is just above the neck of the bottle in use the tubing clip above the drip chamber is closed; the clamp may be applied as an extra safeguard against air entry. The bottle is unhooked and put alongside the new bottle. All that is needed is to remove the piercing needle from the old bottle and insert it into the new bottle after removing the adhesive strip that protects the sterile bung. If the strip has been removed, the area is first swabbed with an antiseptic solution. The needle must not be allowed to touch the edge or the outside of either bottle during this procedure. The full bottle is then suspended from the transfusion stand, the tubing clamp opened and the transfusion continued at the prescribed rate.

The disposable blood pack unit made of polyvinyl chloride is being used in some areas. Unfortunately this material has not yet proved wholly resistant to infection, but it has other advantages over the glass container. The chief ones are related to the transfusion of different components of the blood such as platelets, the anti-D factor required in the treatment of haemolytic disease due to Rh incompatibility, and anti-haemophilic globulin. With the use of these blood pack units, blood is taken from the donor and the anti-haemophilic globulin concentrated by a special process into much smaller volumes of blood which can then be given by intravenous injection in preference to transfusion. The components of plasma such as the anti-D factor are removed from the donor at a time when her titre is high. The blood pack unit is then centrifuged and the plasma expressed into a supplementary bag. The venepuncture is kept open by infusion of normal saline until the remaining packed cells are returned to the donor. By this means, the donor is able to give blood more frequently when required. This procedure is known as plasmaphaeresis.

Difficulties and Dangers that may arise during a Transfusion of Blood or Infusion of other Fluid

1. The introduction of large volumes of blood, or any other fluid, into the blood stream can give rise to cardiac and respiratory distress as a result of overloading the circulatory system. This danger is greatest when large quantities of fluid are rapidly introduced, but can occur with a slow transfusion particularly in elderly patients with a weakened heart muscle or chronic anaemia. Signs which should be watched for and reported to the medical officer immediately are, rising pulse rate, laboured breathing, cough, pain in the chest, distended neck veins and oedema. A fluid intake and output chart should always be kept for a patient who is receiving parenteral fluid.

2. Reactions to the transfusion. A severe reaction occurring soon after the transfusion has been started may be due to incompatibility of the blood and haemolysis of the red cells. The symptoms are: shivering and rise of pulse and temperature; the patient may complain of severe pain in the lumbar region. The transfusion

must be stopped at once. There is great danger of renal failure due to the blocking of the renal tubules by haemolysed blood cells with subsequent suppression of urine and uraemia.

Pyrexial reaction due to the introduction of foreign protein into the blood can also give rise to rigors, fever, and an increased pulse rate. The rate of the transfusion should be slowed, or the transfusion may have to be stopped.

3. Thrombosis of the vein is not uncommon. It may be limited in extent and cause little trouble, but if extensive there is considerable pain in the limb and there may be a rise in the patient's temperature. The transfusion may have to be discontinued and a hot application or an evaporating lotion may be ordered for the relief of pain.

4. A haematoma may form at the site of the transfusion, this results from the needle becoming dislodged from the vein and the blood is then extravasated into the surrounding tissues. The transfusion must be stopped and the limb elevated. An injection of hyalase may be given into the swollen area. There is some danger when the swelling occurs on the anterior aspect of the forearm and elbow that the arteries supplying the forearm may be compressed, and careful watch should be kept on the radial pulse and also on the fingers for blueness and coldness.

5. Sepsis may occur at the site of the infusion. This is more liable to occur when a cannula is tied into the vein than with the use of an intravenous needle or polythene tubing.

6. Air embolism is a rare occurrence but one which must be borne in mind. It is prevented by making sure that air is entirely expelled from the tubing before the

transfusion is started and by taking care that the bottle is not allowed to run dry.

The limb into which the transfusion is running should never be raised above the level of the patient's heart; if the bottle should run out air will be sucked in. No form of pressure should be used to push the blood in at a faster rate; if necessary, the level of the bottle may be raised.

The patient may complain of a variety of sensory disturbances—e.g. tingling in the fingers—and may collapse. The immediate treatment is to lower the patient's head.

7. Difficulty in maintaining the flow of blood may be due to one of several causes. The vein may go into spasm. This may be overcome by gently warming the limb or by stroking along the vein above the injection site.

The tubing may become kinked or pressed upon and this possibility should always be borne in mind and careful inspection made.

The needle may become dislodged. An attempt may be made to alter the position of the needle by gently lifting the mount to depress the point. This may be successful, but if the needle has punctured the wall of the vein the transfusion will have to be stopped and if necessary started again using another vein.

An air-lock may block the flow of blood from the bottle. This should not occur if due care is taken to expel all air from the delivery tubing before connecting it to the needle or cannula. If, however, an air-lock should be present the apparatus must be disconnected from the needle and blood allowed to run freely through the tubing before it is again connected to the intravenous needle.

8. Prolonged intravenous infusion, particularly in the elderly, may lead to a confused state due to a shortage of vitamin B. If this is the cause, parenterovite can be administered via the infusion.

Intravenous Therapy in Babies and Children

The kidneys of babies and children are not as physiologically effective as those of adults and they are susceptible to acid base upsets. For this reason intravenous fluids are given with caution and accurate observations are extremely important throughout the infusion. The electrolyte solutions given vary according to the degree of dehydration and the baby's condition. Molar lactate, Hartmann's solution or Ringer-Lactate, a modified Hartmann's solution, are some of those which may be used.

Subcutaneous Infusion

In cases of dehydration, particularly in babies, it is possible to give fluid, usually ½ normal (isotonic) saline or 5 % dextrose via the subcutaneous route either intermittently or continuously and using hyaluronidase (Hyalase) to aid in its more rapid absorption. The main value of this route is that a doctor is not required to administer the fluid, but absorption is not so effective.

Dialysis

The need for dialysis arises in certain cases of acute disturbance in electrolyte and fluid balance of the body, following loss of kidney function and when other measures have been ineffectual.

Where there is too rapid a rise in blood urea and potassium, haemodialysis is more effective than peritoneal dialysis, mainly because the procedure takes less time. This method, however, requires the constant attention of experienced medical, nursing and technical staff as well as expensive and more bulky equipment.

Dialysis works on the principle that if two solutions of different composition are separated by a membrane which is permeable to the small molecules of the contained solutes, these will cross the membrane until their concentration is equal on the two sides. Applied clinically, this means that peritoneal dialysis can occur between the patient's blood and interstitial fluid (containing an excessive amount of waste products) and a specially prepared electrolyte solution (the dialysis fluid) using the peritoneal membrane as the permeable membrane. The equipment is so constructed that as waste products pass into the dialysing fluid it is then removed and replaced by a fresh supply containing electrolytes and other substances in a concentration which will be most effective in drawing off the remaining impurities. In haemodialysis the blood is drawn out of the body and dialysed in a special machine (the artificial kidney) before being returned to the body.

Peritoneal dialysis can be undertaken in a ward, although a side ward is preferable. The equipment consists of a sterile disposable peritoneal catheter with a metal stylet for introduction and a giving set combined with a sterile plastic bag (or bottle) for collection of returning fluid. The dialysing fluid is contained in sterile plastic bags or in bottles. The proprietary equipment supplied by manufacturers gives instructions and diagrams for aid in assembly.

The patient's bladder is emptied and the anterior abdominal wall prepared as for surgery; the semi-recumbent position is usually adopted. Under a local anaesthetic the catheter is introduced into the peritoneum slightly below the umbilicus in the mid line. If an incision has been made, a skin suture may be required. The appropriate clips are adjusted. The warmed dialysing fluid is then run in to the peritoneal space as fast as it will go, taking about 10 minutes. Most patients will tolerate two litres. The fluid remains in the peritoneal sac for roughly 20 to 30 minutes before the clips are organized to allow it to run out into the collecting bag. Some doctors advise a firm abdominal binder to facilitate drainage. The drainage period should be limited to a maximum of 40 minutes and it is usual for the volume of fluid run out to be less than that run in during the early stages. With later exchanges a negative fluid balance is soon achieved. Failure to drain off the fluid once established may lead to systemic overloading and/ or pulmonary oedema. Blood pressure and fluid balance recordings must therefore be kept throughout. Defects in drainage can arise from catheter blockage from deposition of fibrin. This may be controlled by adding 500 mg of heparin per litre of dialysing fluid, hourly if necessary. Microscopy and culture of the fluid may be ordered and some doctors prefer the addition of an antibiotic as a safeguard against infection. Protein content must also be checked and plasma may be ordered if the blood pressure falls.

Physiotherapy plays an important part in the prevention of pulmonary complications. Good nursing care, support and observations, together with aseptic technique throughout, add to the safety and effectiveness of this treatment.

6. Administration of Dangerous and Scheduled Drugs

Acts of Parliament control the supply and administration of many drugs. Most hospitals have supplemented the statutory requirements by additional rules. All drugs have an official name and it is recommended that this is used but many are marketed by different firms each giving the drug a proprietary name. The Acts of particular concern to nurses are:

The Dangerous Drugs Act

This Act concerns drugs which may give rise to addiction or dependence. They are commonly known as 'D.D.A.s' and include for example:

Opium and its derivatives such as papaveretum (Omnopon), morphine, Nepenthe, diamorphine (heroin) cocaine, pethidine, methadone.

Their container labels are marked D.D.A. In hospital they must be kept in a locked cupboard used *solely* for Dangerous Drugs. The key must be kept on the person of the sister or nurse in charge of the ward or department. The drugs are ordered in a special printed book with carbon copies and a receipt must be signed when they are delivered to the ward. The original requisition is kept in the pharmacy for two years. The custody of the drugs is the responsibility of the sister or her appointed deputy but the cupboard and records may be inspected at any time by the hospital pharmacist or a senior member of the nursing staff.

In most hospitals the regulations for administration

follow a meticulous routine whether the Kardex or similar system operates or whether the prescription is written on the patient's bed ticket or notes.

Two nurses (one of whom is State Registered or an experienced Enrolled Nurse) check the prescription for:

The date.	The patient's full name.
The drug.	The dose.
The route.	The time of administration.
The doctor's signature.	

The remaining ampoules or tablets are checked and recorded.

Once the drug has been drawn into the syringe, the details are checked once more with the prescription.

The patient's identity and the administration of the drug are checked by both nurses at the patient's side and both sign the Dangerous Drugs Record Book immediately afterwards.

Many hospitals require the prescription sheet or Kardex to be signed also, with the time of administration added if necessary.

No cancellation, obliteration or alteration is permitted, corrections being made by way of marginal note signed and witnessed.

The Pharmacy and Poisons Act

This Act is concerned with a large range of potentially dangerous or toxic drugs divided into 17 sections known as Schedules, each subject to special regulations mostly involving the pharmacist. The nurse is chiefly concerned with Schedules 1 and 4.

The container of the drug must be labelled with a distinguishing mark or other indication which shows that it must be stored in a locked cupboard, reserved solely for poisons and other dangerous substances, but separately from the dangerous drugs. The common practice in hospitals is for the Dangerous Drugs cupboard to be contained within this cupboard, each having its own key. Many of the cupboards are lighted from within and a red light indicates that the door is open. If a ward drug trolley is used, it takes the form of a lockable container which must be securely parked when not in use either in a lockable cupboard or by securing to a wall or floor.

Examples of Schedule 1 Drugs are:

Atropine, hyoscine, digoxin, cyclophosphamide, and barbiturate compounds. These are ordered in a separate book from the D.D.A. drugs and are signed for on receipt.

Examples of Schedule 4 Drugs are:

Chloral hydrate, ergometrine and chloral mixture.

These drugs are potentially harmful and most hospitals adopt a scheme of checking for administration and recording for stock balance.

The Therapeutic Substances Act

This Act is concerned with substances often subject to the same restrictions as poisons. Examples are antibiotics, insulin, corticosteroids, vaccines, antitoxins and anticoagulants. Some of these drugs need to be stored in a refrigerator. The same pattern of checking and recording may apply as for the scheduled drugs.

Anticoagulant drugs are usually ordered by the pathologist, according to the percentage of prothrombin, on a special 'Anticoagulant Therapy' form, which is then signed by the nurse giving the drug.

Poisons which are for external use must be contained in a ribbed or fluted bottle which is distinguishable by touch and they should be stored in a cupboard reserved solely for poisons and other dangerous substances. For safety poisons for internal and external use are stored separately.

7. The Classification of Drugs

Anabolic agents. Tissue building male sex hormones prescribed to increase the weight in patients suffering from wasting diseases or osteoporosis, e.g. methandienone (Dianabol), norethandrolone (Nilevar), nandrolone decanoate (Deca-Durabolin). (See Testicular hormones, p. 88.)

Anaesthetics. Drugs which produce insensibility to pain, either by their general action causing loss of consciousness or by local action paralysing the nerve supply in the area. Examples of general anaesthetics are nitrous oxide, halothane (Fluothane) and propanidid (Epontal), given by inhalation, and thiopentone sodium (Pentothal), given by intravenous injection. Examples of local anaesthetics are lignocaine hydrochloride and cinchocaine hydrochloride (Nupercaine).

Analeptics. Drugs which stimulate the nervous system: nikethamide (Coramine), bemegride (Megimide), amiphenazole (Daptazole) and methylamphetamine (Methedrine).

Analgesics. Drugs which relieve pain, e.g. acetylsalicylic acid (Aspirin), pethidine, morphine.

Antacids. Drugs which neutralize the acidity of the gastric juice, e.g. magnesium trisilicate, magnesium carbonate.

Anthelmintics. Drugs used to destroy or expel intestinal parasites, e.g. extract of male fern, piperazine phosphate (Antepar), dithiazanine iodide (Telmid).

Antibiotics. Chemical substances produced from living organisms or synthetically which either inhibit the growth of or destroy other organisms, e.g. penicillin, streptomycin.

Anticholinesterases. Drugs which inhibit the enzyme cholinesterase thereby allowing acetylcholine to accumulate at the nerve endings and restore normal muscle tone. These drugs are used mainly by anaesthetists to reverse the action of drugs used during surgery to produce muscle relaxation, e.g. D-tubocurarine (Tubarine). They may also be used in the treatment of myasthenia gravis and glaucoma and in cases of poisoning from certain agricultural insecticides.

Anticoagulants. Drugs which prevent blood from clotting in the blood vessels, e.g. heparin, dicoumarol, phenindione (Dindevan).

Anticonvulsants. Drugs which reduce the likelihood of abnormal brain rhythms causing convulsions, e.g. phenytoin sodium (Epanutin), Tridione and phenobarbitone.

Antidepressants. Drugs which relieve depression in depressive illnesses, e.g. imipramine (Tofranil) and amitriptyline (Tryptizol). (See also monoamine oxidase inhibitors.)

Antihistamines. Drugs which neutralize the effects of histamines, chiefly used for the treatment of angioneurotic oedema, urticaria and hay fever, e.g. mepyramine maleate (Anthisan) and promethazine hydrochloride (Phenergan), promethazine chlorotheophyllinate (Avomine). These drugs are also used to prevent vomiting following anaesthesia or in travel sickness.

Antipyretics. Drugs which reduce body temperature in fever, e.g. acetylsalicylic acid, quinine.

Antiseptics. Chemical substances which inhibit growth and reproduction of living micro organisms. These may be referred to as bacteriostatics.

Antispasmodics (Spasmolytics). Drugs relieving spasmodic contraction of involuntary muscles, e.g. atropine sulphate, glyceryl trinitrate tablets, Pro-Banthine.

Antithyroid drugs. Drugs which interfere with the production of thyroxine by the thyroid gland, e.g. methyl and propyl thiouracil, Neo-Mercazole.

Antitoxins. Chemical substances which neutralize bacterial toxins. (See also Toxoids and Sera.)

Aperients. Drugs which stimulate intestinal activity, e.g. senna, magnesium sulphate, bisacodyl (Dulcolax).

Bronchial dilators. Drugs which cause relaxation of bronchial smooth muscle which increases vital capacity. They are given in the form of aerosol sprays for inhalation, sub lingually or by injection, e.g. ephedrine, isoprenaline, aminophylline.

Carminatives. Drugs which expel gas and relieve distension in the gastro-intestinal tract, e.g. magnesium carbonate mixture, oil of peppermint.

Contraceptives. The contraceptive pill, or 'The Pill' as it is commonly known, is used in the prevention of pregnancy by inhibiting ovulation, e.g. Minovlar and Norinyl. (See also Hormones.)

Cytotoxics. Substances which act as a poison to certain living cells. Used in the treatment of malignant disease to destroy neoplastic cells, e.g. Cyclophosphamide

(Endoxana), busulphan (Myleran), chlorambucil (Leuk-eran).

Disinfectants. Chemical substances which when used at a prescribed strength for a specific period of time will kill specified micro organisms, e.g. Sudol, chlorhexidine (Hibitane), glutaraldehyde solution (Cidex). See p. 94.

Diuretics. Drugs which increase the output of urine, e.g. cyclopenthiazide (Navidrex-k), chlorothiazide (Saluric), frusemide (Lasix).

Emetics. Drugs which cause vomiting, e.g. zinc sulphate, apomorphine hydrochloride, common salt.

Expectorants. Drugs increasing secretion from the bronchi, e.g. potassium iodide, ammonium carbonate, ipecacuanha.

Fertility drugs. Drugs which increase the output of pituitary gonodotrophins which stimulate the maturation and endocrine activity of the ovarian follicle and the subsequent development of the corpus luteum, e.g. clomiphene citrate (Clomid).

Hypnotics and sedatives. Drugs which induce sleep, e.g. amylobarbitone sodium (Sodium Amytal), butobarbitone (Soneryl), methaqualone (Mandrax).

Hypotensives. Drugs which lower the blood pressure, e.g. propanolol (Inderal), pentolinium (Ansolysen), guanethidine sulphate (Ismelin).

Monoamine oxidase inhibitors. Drugs which act by causing amines normally present in the brain stem (e.g. noradrenaline) to accumulate, thus preventing certain depressive illnesses, e.g. phenalzine (Nardil), isocarboxazid (Marplan), iproniazid (Marsilid). MAO inhibitors have many other biochemical actions too when taken in conjunction with other drugs, alcohol or certain foods, e.g. strong cheese or bananas. Advice must be sought in relation to the patient's diet and other drugs when MAO drugs are being administered.

Muscle relaxants. Drugs used, usually in combination with anaesthetics, to produce complete muscle relaxation which is independent of the depth of anaesthesia, e.g. tubocurarine chloride, Scoline.

Mydriatics. Drugs which dilate the pupil of the eye, e.g. atropine, homatropine.

Myotics. Drugs which contract the pupil, e.g. physostigmine, pilocarpine.

Narcotics. Drugs which act as powerful hypnotics and also as analgesics, e.g. morphine sulphate, papaveretum (Omnopon), pethidine.

Purgatives. (See Aperients.) Drugs which stimulate bowel action, usually applied to those which have a drastic action.

Sera. Serum is prepared from the blood of human beings who have previously suffered from the disease or from animals, usually horses, who are given a vaccine or toxoid to stimulate the production of the appropriate antibodies or antitoxins. Serum from this blood is then used to give protection from specific diseases when the need is urgent. This form of passive immunity can be provided in a matter of minutes but lasts for a period of weeks only since the serum contains proteins foreign to the human body. These can cause severe reactions in susceptible people. Sera may be used to speed protection in the following diseases: anthrax, botulinus, gas gangrene, rabies and german measles. (In persons susceptible to anti-tetanus serum an ovine serum is now available (obtained from sheep).) See p. 73.

Stimulants. (See Analeptics.) Also describes 'tonics' which stimulate the secretions of the gastric mucosa aiding digestion and improving appetite, e.g. gentian, nux vomica and its alkaloid, strychnine.

Toxoids. Liquids containing treated toxins which when introduced into the body stimulate active immunity against certain specific infections caused by bacterial toxins, e.g. diphtheria and tetanus. For persons susceptible to anti-tetanus toxoid a human anti-immunoglobulin is available. See p. 73.

Tranquillizers. Drugs which reduce nervous tension, e.g. promazine hydrochloride (Sparine), chlopromazine (Largactil), chlordiazepoxide (Librium).

Vaccines. Suspensions of dead, living or attenuated micro-organisms or their toxins which when introduced into the human body stimulate active immunity against a specific infection. Diseases against which vaccination gives protection include: smallpox, typhoid fever (T.A.B.), tuberculosis (B.C.G.), poliomyelitis, tetanus, cholera, whooping cough and measles. (See Immunization table.)

8. Pharmaceutical Preparations

Capsules. Drugs, usually either oily or nauseous preparations, enclosed in gelatine envelopes, e.g. librium, halibut-liver oil.

Collodions. Solutions of cellulose in alcohol and ether used as protective coating on the skin and over small dressings, e.g. flexible collodion, salicyclic acid collodion.

Creams. Semi-solid emulsions, usually made up with distilled water or liquid paraffin, for external application, e.g. zinc oxide, hydrocortisone.

Ear-drops. For application to the external auditory meatus, e.g. sodium bicarbonate, cerumol.

Elixirs. Strong extracts of drugs usually made up with syrup and flavouring agents such as liquorice, e.g. cascara sagrada.

Emulsions. Colloidal suspensions of one liquid in another, usually an oil or fat and water, e.g. cod-liver oil, liquid paraffin.

Eye-drops. Sterile preparations for instillation into the eye—e.g. cocaine, antibiotic. Mydriatic eye-drops dilate the pupil, e.g. atropine sulphate. Miotic eye-drops constrict the pupil, e.g. pilocarpine, eserine.

Eye lotions. Usually dispensed with instructions to dilute with an equal quantity of warm water to form a lotion isotonic with the lacrimal secretion and therefore non-irritating, e.g. boric acid, zinc sulphate compound.

Glycerins. Drugs for local application made up in glycerin, e.g. glycerin and ichthyol.

Inhalations. Preparations, commonly made up with industrial alcohol, of drugs to be added to hot water from which the patient inhales vapour, e.g. menthol, tincture of benzoin co.

Irrigations. Solutions, commonly antiseptic or astringent, to be diluted with warm water for application to a cavity, such as the vagina or the bladder, e.g. hibitane 1 in 5,000, normal saline.

Linctuses. Preparations of drugs made up with a syrup base and flavouring agents, used as a cough sedative and intended to be sipped from a spoon, e.g. codeine linctus.

Liniments. Oily preparations, to be applied externally and locally, e.g. methyl salicylate.

Mixtures. Liquid preparations of drugs in water usually containing a number of ingredients, e.g. magnesium trisilicate, kaolin.

Nasal sprays. Water solutions of drugs to be applied to the nasal cavity with an atomizer, e.g. adrenaline, amethocaine.

Ointments. Drugs mixed with fatty substances, such as lanolin or soft paraffin, for external application, e.g. hydrocortisone, resorcinol.

Paints. Fluid preparations, often of a slightly sticky nature, to be applied locally, e.g. iodine compound (Mandl's paint).

Pessaries. Solid preparations usually with a glycerin base containing drugs intended to act locally in the vagina, e.g. nystatin.

Pills. Solid preparations of drugs formed into small balls and often sugar coated, e.g. digitoxin.

Poultices. Drugs incorporated in a soft paste to be warmed and spread on a flannel or cotton backing and applied locally, e.g. kaolin.

Powders. Preparations of drugs in powder form to be mixed with, or swallowed with, water, e.g. compound effervescent (Seidlitz powder), magnesium trisilicate.

Sprays. Drugs incorporated into a pressurized pack to produce very fine droplets, e.g. nobecutane, antibiotic.

Suppositories. Preparations of drugs incorporated in a cocoa butter or glycerin base for insertion into the rectum, e.g. glycerin, aminophylline.

Tablets. Preparations of drugs powdered and compressed, e.g. acetylsalicylic acid (aspirin), butobarbitone (Soneryl).

9. Factors affecting the Dosage of Drugs

The dosage of a drug is modified by certain conditions such as:

Age. Young children can tolerate relatively large doses of some drugs, and react strongly to very small doses of others, notably opium preparations and barbiturates. Dosage for infants and children is usually calculated on the basis of the body-weight, or on a percentage basis related to age. Barbiturates may give rise to confusion in some elderly patients, particularly those over 65 years.

Diet. See monoamine oxidase inhibitors (p. 61).

Disease. The action of any drug may be modified by the disease present, for example, in renal and liver failure drugs are excreted at a slower rate than normal and therefore smaller doses may be given.

Cumulative action. Certain drugs, if taken continually for any length of time, tend to accumulate in the body and may produce harmful effects—e.g. digitalis and large doses of chlorpromazine (Largactil) when prescribed for patients with mental illness.

Idiosyncrasy. Some persons show symptoms of poisoning when given minute doses of certain drugs—e.g. iodine, iron dextran/Imferon, bromides. Even applications of lotions may produce toxic symptoms—e.g. iodine, turpentine.

Tolerance. The opposite of idiosyncrasy, for the individual can tolerate much larger doses than a normal person: this can be natural, or acquired by prolonged use of the drug—e.g. opium, alcohol, arsenic.

Sensitivity reaction. A dramatic response to a drug, such as vomiting, rash, etc. Often associated with administration of serum or penicillin, particularly in patients with a history of asthma.

Habit. Persons who are habitually under the influence of a drug may require larger doses than is usual—e.g. opium.

Race. Coloured races generally tolerate larger doses than white races.

Method of administration. Hypodermic and intramuscular doses are usually smaller, rectal doses larger, than the dose of the same drug given by mouth. Intravenous administration is the fastest route for absorption of a drug.

10. Dosage Table of some Drugs in Common Use

Approved and Proprietary Names	*Dose**
Acetysalicylic acid (Aspirin)	0·3 to 1 g
Adrenalin	1 : 1,000 soln. 0·2 to 0·5 ml s.c.
Ammonium chloride	0·3 to 4 g daily
Amyl nitrite (by inhalation)	0·12 to 0·3 ml
Amylobarbitone (Amytal)	100 to 200 mg
Antibiotics, see p. 74	
Atropine sulphate	0·25 to 2 mg s.c., i.m. or i.v.
Benzhexol (Artane)	2 to 20 mg daily
Benztropine (Cogentin)	0·5 to 6 mg daily
Benthanidine sulphate (Esbatal)	30 mg daily initially—adjust according to response
Bismuth carbonate mixture	0·6 to 2 g
Busulphan (Myleran)	maintenance dose 0·5 to 2 mg daily
Butobarbitone (Soneryl)	60 to 200 mg
Calcium gluconate Calcium lactate }	1 to 5 g according to response
Carbachol	0·25 to 0·5 mg s.c.
Carbimazole (Neo-Mercazole)	Initial dose 30 to 60 mg Maintenance dose 5 to 20 mg
Chloral hydrate mixture	0·3 to 2 g
Chloroquine sulphate	400 mg weekly for malaria
Chlordiazepoxide (Librium)	10 to 100 mg daily
Chlorothiazide (Saluric)	0·5 to 1 g daily
Chlorpormazine hydrochloride (Largactil) Psychiatric purposes	25 to 50 mg oral or i.m. 75 to 1,000 mg daily
Chlorthalidone (Hygroton)	50 to 100 mg daily
Cholinetheophyllinate (Choledyl)	0·4 to 1·6 g daily
Codeine phosphate	10 to 60 mg
Cold-liver oil	4 to 12 ml
Cortisone, see p. 84	
Diamorphine hydrochloride	5 to 10 mg s.c. or i.m.
Diazepam (Valium)	6 to 40 mg
Dichloralphenazone (Welldorm)	0·5 to 2 g as a single dose
Dicoumarol	50 to 300 mg according to prothrombin activity
Digoxin (Lanoxin)	0·25 to 0·75 mg daily maintenance dose

* Unless otherwise stated, the drugs are given in capsule or tablet form.

Approved and Proprietary Names	*Dose*
Dimenhydrinate (Dramamine)	50 to 100 mg
Diphenhydramine (Benadryl)	0·5 mg lozenges
Domiphen bromide (Bradasol)	75 mg daily
Ephedrine hydrochloride	15 to 60 mg
Ergometrine maleate	0·5 to 1 mg
Frusemide (Lasix)	40 to 120 mg daily
Gallamine (Flaxedil)	40 mg per ml i.v.
Glutethimide (Doriden)	250 to 500 mg
Glycerol trinitrate (Sustac)	0·5 to 1 mg
Guanethidine (Ismelin)	Initially 10 to 20 mg Maximum 300 mg
Halibut-liver oil	0·2 to 0·5 ml
Heparin	5,000 to 15,000 units i.v. or i.m.
Isoprenaline (Aleudrin)	5 to 20 mg sublingually
Levallorphan	0·2 to 2 mg
Lugol's iodine (iodine and potassium iodide solution)	0·1 to 1 ml in milk
Magnesium sulphate	5 to 15 g
Mecamylamine hydrochloride (Inversine)	2·5 gradually to maximum of 60 mg
Meprobamate (Equanil)	400 to 1,200 mg daily
Metaraminol tartrate (Aramine)	0·5 to 5 mg i.v. 2 to 10 mg i.m.
Methadone hydrochloride (Physeptone)	5 to 10 mg
Methyldopa (Aldomet)	0·5 increasing to 3 g daily
Metronidazole (Flagyl)	200 to 600 mg daily
Morphine	10 to 20 mg
Nitrazepam (Mogadon)	10 mg
Nitrofurantoin (Furadantin)	200 to 600 mg daily
Noradrenalin (Levophed)	1 in 2,000 solution (amount to be given per minute assessed in each individual case)
Orphenadrine (Disipal)	150 to 400 mg daily
Para-aminosalicylic acid (P.A.S.) see p. 76	
Paracetamol (Panadol)	0·5 to 4 g daily
Paraffin, liquid	10 to 30 ml
Paraldehyde	orally and i.m. 5 to 10 ml rectally 15 to 30 ml diluted
Pentazocine hydrochloride (Fortral)	25 to 100 mg
Pentobarbitone (Nembutol)	100 to 200 mg
Pethidine	50 to 100 mg
Phenelzine (Nardil)	15 to 45 mg daily
Phenindione (Dindevan)	50 to 100 mg according to prothrombin activity
Phenobarbitone	30 to 350 mg
Phenoxybenzamine hydrochlor. (Dibenyline)	10 to 20 mg initially

Approved and Proprietary Names   *Dose*

Phenylbutazone (Butazolidin)	200 to 400 mg
Phenytoin (Epanutin)	50 to 200 mg according to need
Piperazine phosphate (for threadworms)	1 to 2 g
Piperazine phosphate and senna (Pripsen)	10 g
Potassium citrate mixture	2 to 10 g daily
Potassium iodide expectorant mixture	250 to 500 mg
Prednisone	
Prednisolone } see p. 85	
Procainamide hydrochloride (Pronestyl)	orally 500 mg to 1 g daily
Propantheline (Pro-Banthine)	15 mg before each meal
Promethazine hydrochloride (Phenergan)	20 to 50 mg
Proguanil hydrochloride (Paludrine)	prophylactic dose 100 mg daily
Propranalol (Inderal)	30 to 120 mg daily 3 to 10 mg i.v.
Quinalbarbitone (Seconal)	100 to 200 mg
Quinidine sulphate	600 mg to 3 g daily
Reserpine (Serpasil) Hypertension Tranquilizer	0·25 to 0·5 mg daily 5 to 10 mg
Sal volatile (aromatic spirits of ammonia)	1 to 5 ml
Sodium bicarbonate	1 to 5 g
Sodium salicylate mixture	5 to 10 g daily for acute rheumatism
Spironolactone (Aldactone)	50 to 200 mg daily
Sulphonomides, see p. 78	
Sulphone compounds, see p. 79	
Suxamethonium chloride (Scoline)	0·4 to 2 ml i.v. according to need
Tetranicotinoylfructose (Bradilan)	1 g daily adjusted to response
Theophylline with enthylene-diamine (Aminophylline)	0·1 to 0·5 g i.v. or i.m.
Thyroxine sodium	0·05 to 0·3 mg daily

11. Abbreviations in Prescriptions

Latin abbreviations are gradually being replaced by English versions which are considered safer. Where the Kardex or similar prescription sheets are used, they a unnecessary. As the nurse may still meet latin, a selective list is given below.

Abbreviation	Latin	English
aa	ana	of each (i.e. equal parts)
a.c.	ante cibum	before food
ad lib.	ad libitum	as much as desired
aq.	aqua	water
b.i.d. (b.d.)	bis in die	twice a day
c.	cum	with
dil.	dilutus	diluted
fl.	fluidium	fluid
mitt.	mitte	send
M.	misce	mix
N.B.	nota bene	note well
o.m.	omni mane	every morning
o.n.	omni nocte	every night
p.c.	post cibum	after food
p.r.n.	pro re nata	as occasion arises (repeat when required)
q.d. (q.i.d.)	quater in die	four times daily
q.h.	quartis horis	every four hours
s.o.s.	si opus sit	if the occasion arises (a single dose)
ss. (*fs.*)	semis	a half
stat.	statim	immediately
t.d. (t.i.d.)	ter in die	thrice daily
t.d.s.	ter die sumendus	to be taken three times a day

12. Vaccination and Immunization

An Example of a Vaccination and Immunization Schedule as used in the U.K.

Approximate age*	Prophylactic	Date given
6 months	Diphtheria/Tetanus/ Whooping Cough/ and Oral Polio (First Dose)	
8 months	Diphtheria/Tetanus/ Whooping Cough and Oral Polio (Second Dose)	
12–14 months	Diphtheria/Tetanus/ Whooping Cough and Oral Polio (Third Dose)	
15 months	Measles	
16 months	Smallpox	
5 years or school entry	Diphtheria/Tetanus and Polio	
10–13 years	B.C.G.	
15–19 years or on leaving school	Polio Tetanus Smallpox revaccination	

* The ages shown are intended as a guide.

Immunization is also available for certain individuals at risk against the following diseases: rubella (German measles), influenza, rabies or mumps.

It is also available for those travelling to areas where they may encounter diseases not prevalent in their own country, for example: yellow fever, cholera, typhoid and para typhoid fevers, plague and various rickettsial infections.

13. Chemotherapeutic and Antibiotic Agents

Chemotherapeutic drugs, which include the antibiotics, are a class of chemical substances which combat pathogenic organisms in the living tissue of the host. The action of the drug may be bacteriostatic—i.e. preventing the multiplication of bacteria and so enabling the body's defences to combat the infection satisfactorily; or bactericidal, that is, the drug will kill invading organisms. Most chemotherapeutic agents are selective in action, being effective against certain organisms but not all; therefore one factor in successful treatment is the choice of drug.

Antibiotics

This term is used to describe chemotherapeutic substances which are produced by living organisms, or synthetically.

Penicillin. The first and still the most widely used of the antibiotics is penicillin, produced from the mould *Pencillium notatum.*

Penicillin is effective against a number of common organisms including streptococci, staphylococci, pneumococci and gonococci. It is free from toxic side-effects and can be given in very large doses, but some people develop a sensitivity which is manifested by allergic reactions, such as urticaria and even anaphylactic shock. For this reason patients should be asked if they have had previous penicillin treatment, and if thought necessary they should be given a small test dose. Penicillin has one other important disadvantage and that is the development of resistant strains of bacteria, particularly of *Staphylococcus aureus*, which produce an enzyme, penicillinase, which inactivates penicillin. Four main forms of penicillin are in general use:

(1) Benzyl penicillin (penicillin G), a crystalline, soluble form which is quickly absorbed into the blood stream when given by intramuscular injection. Dosage is in the order of 500,000 units to 1 mega unit 4-hourly.

(2) Procaine penicillin which is slowly absorbed and therefore the effect is more prolonged than that of penicillin G. *Dosage*, 500,000 to 1,000,000 units twice daily by intramuscular injection.

(3) Phenoxymethylpenicillin (Penicillin V) and phenethicillin (Broxil) which are unaffected by the acid gastric juice and can therefore be given by mouth. *Dosage*, Penicillin V, 60 to 300 mg by mouth, 4- to 6-hourly. Broxil, 150 to 250 mg by mouth, 4- to 6-hourly.

Substances which hinder the excretion of penicillin and therefore help to maintain the level of the drug in the blood may be given with penicillin. Caronamide and probenecid (Benemid) are two examples of such substances. A successor to methicillin is cloxacillin (Orbenin), which can also be given orally. Dosage 1·5 to 3 g daily.

(4) Ampicillin (Penbritin) is an important broad-spectrum penicillin and may be given by injection or orally.

Penicillin is now seldom used as a local application, although it may be employed in extensive burns, as this method is particularly liable to produce sensitivity to the drug.

Streptomycin. Derived from another mould, *Strepto-myces griseus*. Its main use is in the treatment of all forms of tuberculosis. Resistant strains of *Mycobacterium tuberculosis* are, however, readily produced. The combination of streptomycin with P.A.S. and isoniazid markedly reduces this tendency. Cycloserine and viomycin are two alternative antibiotics which may be given if drug resistance to streptomycin develops. Dosage 0·5 to 0·75 g daily.

Tetracyclines. A group of antibiotics derived from varieties of streptomyces. They are described as 'broad spectrum' antibiotics since they are effective against a wide range of bacteria and also a few viruses and the rickettsiae which cause typhus fever. They are liable to produce some uncomfortable side-effects such as a sore tongue, fungal infection of the mouth and diarrhoea; to combat these a vitamin B preparation is often administered at the same time. The four varieties of tetracycline are:

(1) Chlortetracycline (Aureomycin), *dosage* 250 mg 4-hourly, by mouth.
(2) Tetracycline (Achromycin), *dosage* as above.
(3) Oxytetracycline (Terramycin), *dosage* as above.
(4) Demethylchlortetracycline (Ledermycin), *dosage* 300 mg twice daily.

Chloramphenicol. This drug was originally derived from a form of streptomyces but is now prepared synthetically. Its chief uses are in the treatment of typhoid fever and meningitis. It is effective against a number of organisms but has the disadvantage of depressing the formation of white blood cells if given in large doses, and for this reason its use has been restricted.

Erythromycin. The most active and most widely used of a group of antibiotics all derived from a type of streptomyces and which includes carbomycin, oleandomycin, spiramycin and novobiocin. Erythromycin has a particular use in staphylococcal infections which have proved resistant to penicillin, although resistant strains to this drug can also be produced. *Dosage*, 200 to 500 mg 6-hourly, by mouth.

The polymixins are a group obtained from cultures of the *Bacillus polymyxa*. Polymixin B is effective against infection with *Pseudomonas pyocyanea*, but has the disadvantage of exerting a toxic effect on the kidneys. *Dosage*, 60 mg 4-hourly by intramuscular injection. In cases of *Pseudomonas pyocyanea* meningitis the drug is given intrathecally, 5 to 10 mg in 1 ml of normal saline solution.

Nystatin. Also derived from streptomyces, Nystatin is used as a local application for fungal infections of the skin and mucous membranes.

Griseofulvin (Fulcin) obtained from a variety of penicillium mould is effective against fungal infections of skin, hair and nails. *Dosage*, 250 mg 6-hourly, by mouth.

Cephalosporins. This new group of antibiotics is similar in its action to the penicillin group, but it is claimed that cephalosporins can be given to patients who are sensitive to penicillin. They have a broad spectrum of activity similar to that of ampicillin and can be given orally. Dosage 1 g b.d.

Non-absorbable Antibiotics

Under this classification are grouped a number of antiobitics which are either not absorbed or only slightly absorbed from the alimentary tract when given by mouth. Examples of these are neomycin, paromomycin and colistin. They are prescribed in the treatment of certain intestinal infections—e.g. bacillary dysentery, and prior to operations on the intestines in order to reduce the number of intestinal micro-organisms.

Note: A table showing the sensitivity of some common micro-organisms to chemotherapeutic agents is given on p. 156.

The Sulphonamides

The sulphonamides are of value in the treatment of a wide range of infections. They are especially valuable for urinary tract infections involving gram-negative bacteria, for reducing intestinal bacteria before surgery and in the treatment of meningococcal meningitis.

Examples of sulphonamide compounds in general use are:

(1) Sulphadimidine which is effective against a wide variety of infections, including those due to streptococci, pneumococci and meningococci. Since it has a low toxicity it is one of the most generally useful of the sulphonamide compounds. *Dosage,* initial dose 3 to 4 g, then 1·0 to 1·5 g 6-hourly by mouth.

(2) Sulphadiazine which is particularly useful in the treatment of meningococcal meningitis as it is absorbed into the cerebrospinal fluid. *Dosage,* initial dose 3 to 4 g, then 1·0 to 1·5 g 4-hourly by mouth.

(3) Phthalylsulphathiazole (Thalazole) which is used in the treatment of intestinal infections as it is only slowly absorbed from the alimentary tract. *Dosage* as above.

(4) Sulphamethizole (Urolucosil) which is used for treatment of urinary infections. *Dosage*, 1 g daily .

(5) Sulphamethoxydiazine (Durenate) which is a long acting sulphonamide. *Dosage*, initial dose 1–2 g, then 500 mg daily.

(6) Sulphacetamide (Albucid) which is used for local applications, for example as eye drops in the treatment of conjunctivitis.

Sulphone compounds related to the sulphonamides, of which dapsone and solapsone (Sulphetrone) are examples, are used in the treatment of leprosy. Dapsone solution for injection is prepared in the strength of 0·25g per ml. Dapsone is also dispensed in 100 mg tablets. The dose is prescribed in accordance with the needs of the patient and up to 400 mg may be given twice weekly.

Antituberculosis Drugs (see also p. 76)

Para-aminosalicylic acid (P.A.S.). This drug is only weakly effective against *Mycobacterium tuberculosis*, but used in conjunction with other antituberculosis drugs it helps to prevent the development of drug-resistant strains of the organism. *Dosage*, 12 to 20 g daily by mouth.

2. *Isonicotinic acid hydrazide* (isoniazid, I.N.A.H.). This preparation has an effective action against *Mycobacterium tuberculosis*, but if it is used alone drug resistance can develop quickly. For this reason isoniazid is always used in combination, usually with streptomycin. *Dosage*, 100 to 300 mg daily by mouth. P.A.S. and I.N.A.H. may be given together in a cachet or in the form of granules to be dissolved in milk, when it is known as Inpasade.

3. *Ethambutol*. This drug has a similar action to

D

isoniazid and may be used in its place in combination
with streptomycin. *Dosage*, 300–400 mg daily by mouth
The administration of antituberculosis drugs may be
continued for periods up to 2 years.

The Nitrofurans. This group of drugs is effective
against a wide range of both Gram-positive and Gram-
negative bacteria, including *Staphylococcus aureus*
They are useful in the treatment of infections where the
organism has developed resistance to other chemotherapeutic substances.

Examples of this group are nitrofurantoin (Furadan-
tin) which is excreted in the urine and therefore effective
in the treatment of urinary infections; *dosage* 100 mg by
mouth 4-hourly; furazolidone (Furoxone) which is used
in the treatment of intestinal infections; *dosage*, 100 mg
by mouth 6-hourly; nitrofurazone (Furacin) used as a
local application for wounds and skin conditions.

14. Hormone and Hormone-like Agents

Thyroid Gland Hormones

The thyroid gland manufactures an iodine-containing hormone known as thyroxine which profoundly influences the metabolic processes which convert food substances into energy and into new tissue cells. In childhood it is one of the main factors controlling growth and development. Thyroxine is therefore used in the medical treatment of hypothyroidism which may be congenital (cretinism) or develop in adult life (myxoedema). For many years the standard treatment was to give dried extract of thyroid gland in tablet form by mouth. More recently the pure hormone thyroxine has been extracted.

Preparations at present in use include:

(1) Dried thyroid extract. *Dosage*, 30 to 180 mg by mouth.

(2) Thyroxine sodium. The active principle of the thyroid hormone. *Dosage*, 0·1 to 0·3 mg by mouth.

(3) L-Thyroxine sodium (Eltroxin). A synthetic preparation. *Dosage*, 0·1 to 0·3 mg by mouth.

Anti-thyroid Drugs

In the condition of hyperthyroidism where the thyroid gland produces an excess of thyroxine, various preparations of which the following are examples are used to suppress the activity of the gland.

1. Iodine in the form of potassium iodide or Lugol's solution which is a combination of iodine (5%) and potassium iodide (10%). Iodine diminishes the blood supply in the thyroid gland and temporarily controls

hyperthyroidism; its chief use is as a preoperative treatment given for 10 to 14 days before thyroidectomy is performed. *Dosage*, Potassium iodide 30 to 120 mg by mouth. Lugol's solution, 5 to 15 measured drops by mouth.

2. Propylthiouracil and carbimazole (Neo-Merca-zole) preparations derived from thiourea which inhibit the production of thyroxine.

Dosage, Propylthiouracil, 100 to 400 mg by mouth.
　　　　　Carbimazole, 　　　10 to 40 mg by mouth.

3. Radioactive iodine (I^{131}) is used as a method of diagnosis and for the treatment in selected cases. (See pp. 106, 111, 114.)

Parathyroid Glands

The parathyroid glands situated on the posterior aspect of the thyroid gland secrete a hormone, parathormone which controls the metabolism and blood level of calcium in the body. Over- and under-secretion are generally associated with tumour formation and following thyroidectomy respectively. Hyperparathyroidism is treated by removal of the tumour. Hypoparathyroidism results in tetany and in an increased amount of calcium which is excreted through the renal tract. The treatment is to give calcium orally or by I.V. injection, e.g. calcium gluconate (1–5 g) or lactate.

Adrenal Gland Hormones

Cortical Hormones

The cortex of the adrenal glands produces at least three different types of corticosteroid hormones.

1. Hormones concerned with the regulation of elec-

trolytes and influencing the retention of salt and water and the excretion of potassium.

2. Hormones concerned with the metabolism of proteins and carbohydrates and the conversion and storage of glycogen.

3. Hormones concerned with the building of proteins in the body and also with the development of the secondary sex characteristics.

The main indications for the use of these hormones are as follows:

(a) Replacement therapy in adrenal insufficiency, as for example in Addison's disease (atrophy of the adrenal glands), following bilateral adrenalectomy and in hypopituitarism where the pituitary hormone (ACTH), which stimulates the activity of the adrenal glands, is lacking.

(b) The treatment of a variety of conditions to control their clinical manifestations without, however, curing the underlying pathological process. These conditions include rheumatoid arthritis, asthma, haemolytic and aplastic anaemias, acute leukaemia and the 'collagen diseases' such as disseminated lupus erythematosus and polyarteritis nodosa, and in inflammatory and allergic skin conditions. Where these hormones are given over long periods, side-effects are likely to occur, such as salt and water retention leading to oedema, loss of potassium, hypertension, changes in appearance (the so-called 'moon-face'), mental disturbances and peptic ulcer. A low salt diet with additional potassium may be ordered, and prednisone, a derivative of cortisone, is often used in its place and is liable to cause oedema.

The administration of cortical hormones suppresses the normal activity of the adrenal glands, and therefore these drugs are withdrawn gradually to prevent the occurrence of acute adrenal insufficiency. A patient who is receiving replacement therapy requires a constant and adequate supply of whichever drug is prescribed. The maintenance dose will need to be increased if the patient suffers an intercurrent illness, or if an operation becomes necessary. It is a wise precaution for him to carry a card stating his condition, the drug he is taking and the dosage, in case of sudden illness or accident.

The list set out below gives examples of the most widely used cortical hormones and synthetic substitutes.

Aldosterone. A naturally occurring hormone influencing sodium and water retention and potassium excretion.

Deoxycortone (D.O.C.A.). A synthetic product first used in the treatment of Addison's disease. *Dosage*, 3 to 5 mg by intramuscular injection, or pellets of 50 to 100 mg for subcutaneous implantation and slow absorption.

Fludrocortisone. A synthetic preparation with similar properties to aldosterone. It is used in the treatment of Addison's disease and following bilateral adrenalectomy in addition to cortisone to prevent excessive loss of sodium. *Dosage*, 0·1 to 0·3 mg by mouth.

Cortisone. One of the hormones in group (*b*) above, cortisone is used in the treatment of Addison's disease and other forms of adrenal insufficiency, and also in a variety of disorders for its role in maintaining the essential chemical functions of the tissue cells in times of stress. *Dosage*, cortisone is dispensed in 25 mg tablets, the dosage depends on the type and severity of the condition for which it is prescribed, but is in the order of 50 to 500 mg.

Hydrocortisone. Similar to cortisone but has a wider

range of usefulness. It can be applied to skin and mucous membrane for local effect and also injected into joints in the treatment of rheumatic conditions. Hydrocortisone acetate and hydrocortisone hemisuccinate are the two preparations most commonly used, and can be supplied as a solution for injection and as a cream or ointment for local application. *Dosage*, hydrocortisone sodium succinate 100 mg by intramuscular or intravenous injection.

Prednisone and Prednisolone. Two synthetic substitutes for cortisone. They are about five times as active as the naturally occurring hormones and are given in smaller dosage. In addition to their use as substitutes for cortisone in the conditions mentioned above, these two preparations are also used in the palliative treatment of malignant disease. *Dosage*, both preparations are dispensed in 5 mg tablets.

Medullary Hormones

These hormones produce effects similar to those produced by stimulation of the sympathetic nervous system —i.e. increased heart rate, raised blood pressure and the release of glycogen as fuel for immediate use. In medical practice these substances are used to relieve bronchial spasm in asthma and to counteract anaphylactic reactions.

Adrenaline (epinephrine), used in the treatment of asthmatic attacks, allergic conditions, anaphylaxis, and also locally to control bleeding and with local anaesthetics to slow down the absorption of these agents. *Dosage*, 0·1 to 0·5 mg, 5 to 10 ml of a 1 in 1,000 solution given by hypodermic injection.

Ephedrine has a longer action than adrenaline. Its chief use is in the relief of bronchospasm in asthma. It can be given by mouth. *Dosage*, 15 to 100 mg.

Isoprenaline, a derivative of adrenaline, affects the cardiovascular system by producing tachycardia, but it has a marked action in relieving spasm of the bronchi in asthma. It may be used as an aerosol spray or in the form of tablets to be placed under the tongue and absorbed from the mouth. *Dosage*, for aerosol spray, 1 % solution; for sub-lingual administration 5 to 20 mg.

Pituitary Gland Hormones

Anterior Lobe Hormones

The anterior lobe of the pituitary gland produces a number of hormones which stimulate the activity of other endocrine glands, but there are few pharmaceutical preparations of these hormones.

1. Gonadotrophic hormone, which is obtained from the urine of pregnant women, is available under the name of Antuitrin-S or Pregnyl or clomiphene citrate (Clomid) a non steroidal preparation. It may be used in the treatment of sterility in women and also in cases of undescended testicles in boys. *Dosage*, 500 to 1,000 units by intramuscular injection.

2. Adrenocorticotrophin (ACTH) which stimulates the activity of the cortex of the adrenal glands. This hormone had an important place in treatment of various conditions in which the corticosteroids are effective, but it has the disadvantage of being short-acting and also it must be given by injection. Its use has diminished since the introduction of hydrocortisone and the synthetic preparations, such as prednisone and prednisolone. *Dosage*, 20 to 40 units.

Posterior Lobe Hormones

Posterior pituitary gland hormones influence the retention of fluid, the 'anti-diuretic' hormone, and also have the effects of raising the blood pressure and causing contractions of the uterine muscle. Preparations used in treatment include the following.

Pituitrin, which contains all the posterior lobe hormones. It may be prescribed in the treatment of diabetes insipidus for its anti-diuretic effect, either in the solution of 10 units per ml for injection or as a powder to be used as a snuff. *Dosage*, 5 to 10 units by hypodermic injection, or 5 to 10 mg dried powder to be used as a snuff.

Vasopressin (Pitressin) also used in the treatment of diabetes insipidus. *Dosage*, 5 to 15 units by intramuscular injection.

Oxytocin (Pitocin) stimulates contractions of the uterus and is used in obstetric practice for this purpose, as for example in the treatment of post-partum haemorrhage. It may be used orally or in an intravenous 'drip' form to induce labour. Oxytocin is dispensed in solution containing 10 units per ml. *Dosage*, 0·2 to 5 units by intramuscular injection.

Sex Hormones

The sex hormones are produced by ovarian tissue in the female and testicular tissue in the male.

Ovarian Hormones

Oestrogens. The naturally occurring hormone oestradiol, and synthetic substitutes such as stilboestrol, dienoestrol and ethinyloestradiol, are used in the treatment of menopausal symptoms. They are also used in the treatment of malignant disease of the prostate gland in the male and carcinoma of the breast; in the latter case these hormones are used for women only after the menopause.

Dosage: Oestradiol, 1 to 10 mg by mouth.
Stilboestrol, 0·5 to 2 mg by mouth.
Dienoestrol, 0·1 to 1·5 mg.
Ethinyloestradiol, 0·01 to 1 mg.

Progesterone is produced by the corpus luteum. In medical practice it is used in the treatment of threatened abortion. *Dosage*, 5 to 20 mg by intramuscular injection.

Ethisterone. A derivative of progesterone, can be given by mouth. *Dosage*, 60 to 100 mg by mouth.

'The Pill.' The contraceptive pill is used in the prevention of pregnancy by inhibiting ovulation. Oral contraceptives fall into three groups. One group contains a progestogen and oestrogen in combination. Another group known as the sequential group contains two types of tablet—one containing an oestrogen alone, followed by a combination tablet to complete a course. A third group contains a low dose of progesterone alone in each tablet. This pill has so far proved to be less satisfactory. The pills which fall within the first two groups are taken on specific days related to the period before and after ovulation. Examples are: Minovlar and Norinyl.

Testicular Hormones. Male sex hormones secreted by the testes are responsible for the development and maintenance of the male sexual system. They affect protein metabolism and calcium retention. Testosterone can be used therapeutically in testicular deficiency in the male and also in menstrual disturbances and carcinoma of the breast in the female. They are also used to increase weight in cases of senile osteoporosis and debilitating diseases. Unfortunately when used in female patients, these hormones have a virilizing effect but there are now some testosterone derivatives in use which are able to lessen the virilizing effects. (See also p. 58, Anabolic Agents.) Methyl testosterone can be given by mouth. *Dosage*, 5 to 25 mg daily.

Pancreatic Hormone (Insulin)

Insulin, extracted from the islets of Langerhans in the pancreas, is mainly used in the treatment of diabetes mellitus.

The preparations of insulin at present in use include soluble insulin, which is quick acting and therefore particularly useful in the treatment of diabetic ketosis, in diabetic patients undergoing surgery and in emergencies such as an acute infection occurring in a diabetic patient. It may also be given in combination with the longer acting type of insulin.

Longer Acting Preparations

1. Insulin Zinc Suspensions (IZS) are available in three forms: 'semilente' (IZS Amorphous), 'lente' (IZS) and 'ultralente' (IZS Crystalline). Of these, semi-lente has the shortest period of activity and ultralente the longest.

2. Protamine Zinc Insulin is long acting and is similar to ultralente. It may be given in combination with soluble insulin, which should be drawn up first into the syringe.

3. Globin Zinc Insulin has an intermediate action similar to lente.

4. Isophane Insulin may also be combined with soluble insulin.

Occasionally a patient is allergic to insulin of bovine origin and the purer form which comes from the pancreas of the pig is ordered, e.g. Actrapid or neutral.

Dosage of insulin is 'tailored' to meet the requirements of the individual diabetic patient in relation to the severity of the condition and the diet he needs in order to maintain his health and energy. He is then said to be 'stabilized'.

Insulin should be stored in a cool atmosphere, otherwise it may undergo changes which could produce a reaction in the patient.

Administration of Insulin

The standard strengths of insulin for injection are:

> 20 units in 1 ml (single strength).
> 40 units in 1 ml (double strength).
> 80 units in 1 ml (quadruple strength).

An insulin or 'unit' syringe is generally used. The markings differ according to the manufacturer. It is usually of 2 ml capacity and may be graduated into either:

> (A) 10 divisions to each ml, or
> (B) 20 divisions to each ml.

The ordinary type of 1 or 2 ml syringe can also be used but it is unsuitable for small doses.

Example: Using Insulin (Unit) Syringe

If the insulin dose prescribed is 32 units, then:

> 32 units single strength would be drawn up
>
> or
>
> 16 units double strength would be drawn up
>
> or
>
> 8 units quadruple strength would be drawn up.

Example: Using ordinary syringe with 5 divisions to each ml

> 8 divisions single strength would be drawn up

or

> 4 divisions double strength would be drawn up

or

> 2 divisions quadruple strength would be drawn up.

Anti-diabetic Drugs

All types of insulin must be given parenterally since insulin is destroyed by the gastric juice. The anti-diabetic drugs which are now available for oral administration are not forms of insulin but are compounds derived from the sulphonamides which apparently act by stimulating the islet cells in the pancreas.

Three of the preparations in use at the present time are:

1. *Tolbutamide* (Rastinon) which is rapidly excreted and therefore several doses are required daily. *Dosage*, 0·5 to 3 g by mouth daily in divided doses.

2. *Chlorpropamide* (Diabinese) which is slowly excreted and therefore a single daily dose is usually sufficient. *Dosage*, 100 to 500 mg by mouth daily in a single dose.

3. *Glybenclamide* (Euglucon). *Dosage*, 2·5 to 10 mg daily taken with, or immediately after a meal.

The Liver and the Anti-anaemic Factor

Liver extracts were for many years used in the treatment of macrocytic hyperchromic (or pernicious) anaemia until it was discovered that the actual anti-anaemic factor in these extracts was vitamin B^{12} or cyanocobalamin, which the liver is able to store in considerable quantities. The dosage of cyanocobalamin (Cytamen) for the initial treatment of pernicious anaemia is 100 to 250 micrograms on alternate days for 1 to 2 weeks, then weekly and finally 250 micrograms every 2 or 3 weeks as a maintenance dose. If hydroxocobalamin (Neocytamen) is used the usual maintenance dose is 1,000 micrograms at 2 to 4 weekly intervals. These dosages may vary in relation to the response to treatment and will be higher if there is neurological involvement.

15. Chemical Disinfectants and Antiseptics in General Use

Many drugs which are named as disinfectants are not necessarily bacteriocidal to all living organisms. Before they can be said to sterilize instruments or equipment, they must be used at a prescribed strength for a specific period of time and be in direct contact with the articles to be sterilized, which should be adequately rinsed before use. Unless these principles are applied, chemical disinfection may well prove unreliable. Where any doubt exists, the advice of the bacteriologist should be sought and the suspected organisms named.

It is the practice in most hospitals for the label on the stock bottle of disinfectant or antiseptic to indicate the strength at which the solution should be used and to quote how the required dilution will be made up. The nurse should adhere strictly to these instructions as a lotion used in either too weak or too strong a solution may be potentially harmful to the user, the equipment or to the patient involved. For example chlorhexidine (Hibitane) is used in different strengths and may be in an alcoholic or aqueous solution according to its application.

To avoid painful smarting, spirit-based antiseptics should not come into contact with skin directly after it has been shaved, or with mucous membrane. Iodine in spirit may cause blistering if it is not allowed to evaporate after application to the skin.

Some examples of disinfectants and antiseptics are shown overleaf.

Chemical	Examples of Uses	Strength
Acridines, a group of dyes which include aminacrine, flavine, euflavine, proflavine hemisulphate	Swabbing wounds, aqueous solution Skin antisepsis— alcoholic solution	1 in 1,000 solution
Benzalkonium chloride (Roccal)	Skin antisepsis Disinfection of utensils and linen	1 in 10 solution 1 in 40 solution
Chlorine preparations e.g. Eusol Sodium hypochlorite solution (Milton)	As a dressing or as an irrigating solution for infected or sloughing wounds As above and also for disinfecting feeding utensils, e.g. infants' feeding bottles	0·5 to 2% solution 1 in 80 solution
Chlorhexidine (Hibitane)	Skin and wound antisepsis, or as an irrigating solution or obstetric cream	0·02 to 0·5% in 70% alcohol for skin antisepsis 1 in 5,000 aqueous solution for irrigation
Chloroxylenol (Dettol, Osyl, Roxenol)	Less caustic than phenol or cresol preparations. Used for general disinfection of utensils and linen Antiseptic hand lotion Vaginal douching	1 in 20 solution. For vaginal douching 1 in 40 solution
Cresols, coal tar derivatives (Izal, Cylin, Jeyes' fluid)	Disinfection of excreta and sanitary utensils, linen, local pollution of floors, e.g. with sputum	Excreta, 1 in 10 solution left for 2 hours. Linen, 1 in 160 solution for 12 hours. Mop floors with 1 in 50 solution
Cresol with soap (Lysol, Sudol)	Disinfection of basins and baths after use Preparation of theatre and dressing trolleys before use	Mop with 1 in 20 solution, leave for 5 minutes, rinse thoroughly with hot water Mop with 1 in 120 solution

Chemical	Examples of Uses	Strength
Domiphen bromide (Bradosol)	Skin and wound antisepsis	1 in 2,000 solution
	Disinfection of utensils	1 in 500 solution
Formaldehyde, as a gas or in solution as formalin Paraform tablets	For disinfecting rooms, bedding, books and articles which cannot be heat sterilized without damage. Used in disinfection of rooms, also in sealed containers for disinfection of gum elastic articles, e.g. catheters	
Glutaraldehyde solution (Cidex)	Kills all vegetative organisms after 10 minutes immersion. Particularly recommended for the sterilization of endoscopic and general anaesthetic equipment which is unsuitable for heat treatment. Reservations concern the effectiveness of this disinfectant against the viruses producing hepatitis	When activated (by mixing powder and solution together) the product remains effective for 14 days without replacement
Hexachlorophane soap with Gamophen	Surgical soap containing hexachlorophane for surgical scrubbing and hand washing containing 2% hexachlorophane	
Phisohex, cream contains 3% hexachlorophane	For surgical 'scrubs' and hand washing	
Synthetic phenol (Hycolin)	Cleansing and disinfection of walls, floors and surfaces of dressing trolleys and operating tables	1% solution for general use, 2% solution for surgical instruments

Chemical	Examples of Uses	Strength
Stericol	Thermometers in the ward and surgical instruments	
Hydrogen peroxide	Used for cleaning wounds and cavities, e.g. the mouth. In the presence of organic material liberates oxygen. Is non-poisonous	Stock solutions contain either 10 or 20 volumes of available oxygen. Dilute with water as necessary, for use in 2·5 or 5 volume strength
Iodine	Used for skin antisepsis especially pre-operatively. Is more penetrating than most skin paints, when used on dry skin	2·5 % in 70% alcohol
Povidone iodine (Betadine)	Non staining, for use on skin and mucous membrane	1% solution
Phenol (carbolic acid)	Caustic and poisonous, now largely replaced by less dangerous preparations. May be used for disinfecting excreta, sanitary utensils, crockery, linen, bed macintoshes	For excreta: 1 in 10 solution, for other purposes 1 in 20 or 1 in 40 solution
Savlon A proprietary preparation combining chlorhexidine and cetrimide	Used for cleaning skin, also for burns and wounds Washing hospital equipment and disinfecting linen	1 in 100 solution

16. X–ray Examinations

X-ray examination interpretation is based on shadows, and pathology is recognized by either addition to or subtraction from these shadows. Many hospitals now have television cameras and monitor screens linked to the screening unit and the room need not be so dark as formerly. It is essential to eliminate from the field of investigation any substances likely to cast shadows on the radiograph. A list of some extraneous substances is as follows:

Clothing: silk and artificial silk, buttons, elastic, pins, hair-clips.

Radio-opaque dressings or applications, e.g. those impregnated with iodine, lead lotion, kaolin, etc.

Elastoplast.

Kaolin, Thermogene wool.

Rubber tubes.

Wigs, breast prostheses, dentures and artificial eyes.

Metallic splints except aluminium.

Plaster of paris splints obscure detail, particularly while still wet, but it is usually possible to get a reasonable radiograph of fracture through plaster.

Bowel content and gas cast shadows and obscure detail, which make pathology of the urinary system, coccyx and even lumbar spine difficult to recognize.

Adherence to recognized rules in the preparation of the patient aids the accuracy of the subsequent diagnosis, saves the patient the inconvenience and possible discomfort of a repeated examination, and saves time, labour and cost in the X-ray department. *If there is any doubt as to the correct procedure in any case specific instructions should be sought from the radiologist.* The patient should receive a reasonable explanation of what will be involved in the examination and be told that he may need to spend some considerable time in the X-ray department. Nurses should ensure that patients are both warm and comfortable before leaving the ward.

Examination of the Alimentary Tract

Barium Meal Examination

The contrast medium used for this examination is barium sulphate. Various proprietary preparations are also used.

The object of the preparation is to have the patient's stomach empty at the time when the examination is made. No food or drink is allowed for at least 6 hours prior to the barium meal and many radiologists prefer 12 hours' starvation. No aperient should be given within 24 hours of the examination and any medicine containing heavy metals—e.g. bismuth—should be discontinued for at least two days previously. The examination may extend over a period of 24 hours or 48 hours; no food is usually allowed until the stomach is seen to be empty and no aperients or enemas until the examination is complete.

It is helpful if the patient is able to stand during the examination: therefore if he has been confined to bed for some time he should be allowed to sit out of bed for a day or two and to stand before the visit to the X-ray department.

If the examination is undertaken for investigation of the appendix, an aperient is given 36 hours before the examination begins and no food or drink is allowed for

6 hours before the barium is given. A 'Follow through' examination will be required. After the first examination the patient may have his usual diet but no aperient may be given until the examination is completed.

Barium Enema Examination

The object of the preparation of the patient is to clear the colon of faeces and gas. An aperient is given on the day before the examination and a Dulcolax suppository or rectal washout given prior to the barium enema. Where possible the patient should be encouraged to walk about or move in bed to help in the expulsion of flatus. Light diet is usually allowed on the day of the examination. A film may be required 24 hours after the enema and in this case no aperient or enema should be given until the examination is complete.

Examination of the Gall-Bladder

Cholecystography. The object of the preparation is first to empty the gall-bladder in order that the dye may be concentrated in it, then to encourage the dye-filled gall-bladder to empty before the final films are taken.

An aperient is given 2 days before the examination, the dose required depending on what suits the patient. On the evening prior to the examination, a light meal consisting of non-fatty foods is taken. Permitted are: fresh vegetables cooked without fat, fruit or fruit juices, lean meat, toast or bread, coffee or tea. All fried or fatty foods must be omitted, e.g. milk, butter, eggs or salad dressing. Apart from a small amount of water, nothing else to eat or drink must be taken until after the X-ray examination.

On the night before the examination Biloptin capsules are swallowed with a little water. The dose depends on the size of the patient and may vary between 6 to 12 capsules. It is important that they are swallowed whole and not chewed. Smoking should also be avoided.

After the first films have been taken, a pre-packed fat-containing preparation is given before further films are taken. The instructions issued by the X-ray department may differ from this routine and in some instances, if one dose fails to outline the gall-bladder, two doses may be required.

Biligrafin or Telepaque may also be used to outline the biliary tract. It should be noted that all preparations may produce side effects in some patients, for example, nausea, vomiting or diarrhoea, but Biloptin is thought to produce the least.

Examination of the Urinary Tract

Intravenous Pyelography

The objects of the preparation are to have the bowel empty and to concentrate the urine.

On the first day of the preparation the patient is allowed light diet but fluids are restricted. He should have an aperient in the evening, usually a vegetable laxative is ordered.

On the second day the same preparation is repeated.

On the day of the examination no fluids are allowed for at least 6 hours prior to the X-ray. Light breakfast is allowed. It is very important that the aperient given on the previous evening shall be effective. In order to prevent accumulation of gas in the intestine the patient should if possible be encouraged to walk about. Charcoal biscuits may be given at breakfast and the medical officer may order an injection of prostigmin or pituitary extract.

The patient must empty the bladder immediately before the examination.

The contrast media used for this examination are iodine-containing solutions, e.g. diodone (Uriodone), Contay, Hypaque.

Drip infusion pyelography. In some cases where the blood urea exceeds 100 mg per 100 ml, the doctor may decide to introduce the dye by intravenous drip method as this gives a better concentration. It is not necessary to restrict fluids before this examination.

Retrograde or Instrumental Pyelography

This examination is carried out by injecting a contrast medium, a sterile solution of sodium iodide, into the pelvices of the kidneys by means of ureteric catheters. A cystoscope is first passed and the ureters are then catheterized. Usually about 7 ml of the solution is required to fill the pelvis of the kidney, but the injection is stopped as soon as the patient complains of pain. The strength of the solution used varies; it may be 10, 20 or 30% sodium iodide. (Urografin.)

Straight X-ray of the urinary tract. This examination consists of taking films of the urinary tract without the use of contrast media.

The preparation for retrograde pyelography and for 'straight' X-ray is the same as for intravenous pyelography, except that there is no need to restrict fluid.

Micturating Cystogram

No specific preparation of the patient is required for this examination. A catheter is passed, the bladder emptied and the contrast medium is injected through this until the bladder is moderately full. The catheter is withdrawn and radiographs are taken while the patient is asked first to 'strain' but to hold the urine and then to pass urine into a receptacle provided. This examination may be used in the investigation of stress incontinence in women patients, and of urinary infections in childhood, when reflux of urine from the bladder along the ureters may sometimes be detected.

Examination of the Lumbar Spine, Sacrum and Pelvis

In some cases no preparation of the patient is carried out prior to taking the films, in others the preparation as described for X-ray of the urinary tract may be ordered.

Examination of the Chest

This requires no preparation, unless a bronchogram is to be carried out, beyond the removal of all clothing likely to cast shadows.

Bronchography. The contrast media used in this examination are iodized oil (Lipiodol, Neo-Hydriol) and Dionosil. The medium may be introduced into the bronchi through a special syringe with a curved dropper attached dropping the oil into the trachea via the mouth. A local anaesthetic and spray are required to anaesthetize the pharynx.

An alternative method is to insert a short curved cannula into the trachea through the cricothyroid membrane. This may also be carried out under a general anaesthetic.

Premedication in the form of a sedative drug and also an injection of atropine may be ordered. Usually the patient is not allowed any food within 6 hours of the examination owing to the tendency to vomit. After the examination it is important that the patient should not be allowed any food or drink until the effects of the local anaesthetic have completely disappeared and the cough reflex is re-established. Postural drainage may be ordered before and after the examination.

Examination of the Uterine (Fallopian) Tubes

Salpingography. This examination consists of taking films of the pelvis after the introduction of iodized oil into the uterine tubes. The oil is introduced through an intrauterine nozzle attached to the special syringe used for iodized oil. The same preparation is required as for 'straight' X-ray of the urinary tract. It is not undertaken during menstruation. Pre-medication may be ordered.

Examination of the Brain

Cerebral angiography. This is used to demonstrate the cerebral blood vessels by introducing a contrast medium into the carotid or vertebral arteries. The X-ray films obtained may demonstrate such abnormalities as an aneurysm, a tumour of the brain or a haematoma resulting from a subdural or an extradural haemorrhage. Any one of these may displace an artery from its normal position.

Under a local or general anaesthetic with the use of a special needle, the contrast medium is introduced into the carotid or vertebral artery through a length of plastic tubing. Several films are then taken in different planes.

Encephalography. A lumbar puncture is carried out and a measured quantity of air equal to the amount of cerebrospinal fluid removed is injected into the sub-arachnoid space. This air, being lighter than the cerebrospinal fluid, rises rapidly into the communicating ventricles of the brain. A series of films of the skull is then taken as in ventriculography.

Myelography. This is used to demonstrate any obstruction to the passage of cerebrospinal fluid down the spinal canal, such as a tumour or disc protusion. The procedure is similar to that for encephalography using contrast medium in place of air. If the suspected lesion is in the cervical region the injection is via the cisterna magna as in cisternal puncture.

Ventriculography. X-ray films of the skull are taken after the injection of air into the ventricles of the brain. The procedure involves making trephine holes through the parietal bones, removing cerebrospinal fluid from the ventricles and injecting air. This operation is carried out by the surgeon in the theatre and the usual preparations for any cranial operation are required. The appropriate area of scalp must be shaved and the skin prepared.

The usual reason for the examination is to aid in the diagnosis or location of a brain tumour, and the operation for removal of the tumour is proceeded with at once if the X-ray findings confirm the diagnosis.

These procedures may be followed by severe headache and/or nausea in the patient who may require sedation on return to the ward and bed rest for several hours.

Examination of the Cardiovascular System

Arteriography. With an opaque medium, Hypaque Urografin or Conray, this is used to demonstrate the blood supply to a particular area, for example:

Femoral arteriography. Introduction of an opaque medium via the femoral artery can be used to demonstrate the blood supply to the lower limbs, the kidneys (renal arteriography) and, in pregnancy, the placenta. This method is also used to investigate the left side of the heart.

The patient is prepared for a general anaesthetic or a local anaesthetic may be used. The pubic area is shaved and the skin cleaned. A thin plastic tube or catheter is introduced into the femoral artery with a special needle and passed along the artery to the required position. The contrast medium is then injected and the films taken. Alternatively a narrow beam of radiation about 12 mm ($\frac{1}{2}''$) in width scans down the length of the artery producing a series of films inside a long film holder which is called a cassette.

Cardiac Catheterization (Cardio-angiography). This may be used to detect congenital heart lesions and other types of heart disease. A long opaque catheter is introduced through one of the right arm veins into the right atrium, its course being controlled by a television monitor screen. To demonstrate the left side of the heart, the catheter is introduced via the femoral artery, as in arteriography. Before the contrast medium is injected, the cardiac catheter may be connected to a manometer to record pressures in the heart. Blood samples may be taken through it to assess the oxygen saturation in the various chambers of the heart and great vessels.

For these investigations a local anaesthetic is used for adults, but a general anaesthetic may be required for a child.

Patients should be warned and reassured beforehand about the amount of complicated equipment which will face them on arrival in the X-ray room.

Following arteriography, observation of the site of

the injection in the groin is important and should continue for several hours to avoid the complication of haemorrhage from the femoral artery.

Radioactive Isotopes

Other types of ray are obtained from radioactive substances (radio isotopes) which are used mainly for therapy either from sealed sources such as radon seeds or unsealed sources in liquid form such as radioactive iodine. Unsealed sources may also be used in diagnosis, given in smaller tracer quantities to a patient as a drink or injection, followed by 'scanning' of the part under investigation—for example, the liver, the brain, the circulation or lung function. (See also pp. 111, 112.)

17. The Therapeutic Use of X—rays and Radioactive Substances

X-rays and the radiations from the naturally occurring radioactive elements, such as radium, and from artificially produced radioactive isotopes of certain elements have fundamentally similar properties. They are all forms of energy making up one part of the vast electromagnetic spectrum, propagated in wave formation and able to penetrate materials opaque to visible light. These radiations affect living cells and in sufficient quantities can destroy living tissue. The therapeutic use of radioactive substances is based on the fact that some cells are more readily damaged than others. Rapidly dividing and growing cells are more radiosensitive than older cells, therefore the cells of a rapidly growing malignant tumour can be killed by a dose which, if carefully distributed, produces little if any permanent damage to the surrounding healthy tissues.

Deep X-ray Treatment

This term implies the use of penetrating X-rays produced by the bombardment of a target by electrons travelling at high speed. The source of the energy required for this is high voltage electricity, of the order of 180 to 100,000 kilovolts or higher. This form of treatment is most frequently used in cases of malignant growth, either alone or in combination with surgery.

The majority of the patients require a large dose spread over a period of several weeks in order that a lethal dose can be delivered at the site of the growth without producing either generalized ill-effects or localized damage to the skin and surrounding tissues.

However carefully the scheme of treatment is devised the tissues surrounding the growth are likely to suffer at least some temporary ill-effects and this is especially true of the skin. Therefore great care is required during and for some weeks after the treatment. The skin may be washed with soap and water, but it must be thoroughly dried without the use of vigorous rubbing. Graneodin ointment may be found soothing. If a male patient is receiving treatment to the face or neck, shaving is usually forbidden for a time, although dry shaving with an electric razor is allowed, and the friction of a closely fitting stiff collar should be avoided. Mucous membrane reacts to radiation in much the same way as skin and some temporary damage to mucus secreting cells will occur. If the mouth is included in the treatment area there will be a diminution in the secretion of both saliva and mucus. The patient may be very disinclined to eat on account of the discomfort and pain caused by a dry mouth and must be helped and encouraged as much as possible. Frequent non-irritating fluids to drink and frequent mouth washes will help. If the mouth is painful, lozenges containing a local anaesthetic —e.g. Benzocaine—may be ordered, or aspirin gargles may give relief.

General effects of radiation are not usually marked when divided dosage is used spread over a period of weeks, but were fairly common in the early days of X-ray treatment when a single large dose was used. However, some patients may complain of loss of appetite, nausea, diarrhoea, inability to sleep and general depression. It may be noted that some of these effects may be due to the rapid disintegration of the mass of malignant cells.

Superficial application of X-rays is a method of treatment used in rodent ulcer and skin conditions such as keloid scars, also occasionally in some conditions such as acne, which have proved resistant to other forms of treatment. Treatment is usually planned in collaboration with the dermatologist and specific instructions will be given as to whether or not local applications are to be used at the same time.

Radium

Radium is a naturally occurring element which spontaneously emits radiations of short wave-length. The penetrating radiations, known as gamma rays, are used therapeutically, other radiations from radium, alpha and beta rays are screened off by the metal walls of the radium container. Radium is chiefly used in the form of its salt, radium sulphate, and in the form of the emanation of gas, radon, which is given off from it. The salt is placed in needles, gold 'grains' or into larger containers.

Methods of Application

Surface application. The needles or applicators are embedded in a suitable mould made of Columba paste, Perspex or Stent's dental composition, or may be attached to sorbo rubber or other suitable material which can be accurately applied to the desired area.

Interstitial irradiation. Needles or gold 'grains' are inserted into the tissues.

Cavitary irradiation. Applicators are placed inside natural cavities of the body—e.g. the vagina and cervical canal.

Rules and Precautions in handling Radium

A standard symbol (above) has been adopted to denote the actual or potential presence of radiation and these discs are appropriately placed wherever there is a risk of contamination.

1. Radium needles or containers should never be touched by hand but must always be manipulated with long-handled forceps the handles of which are covered with rubber. When radium is removed from the safe and carried to and from the theatre a lead-lined box with a long carrying handle should be used for its transport.

2. The threading of needles and the preparation of applicators must be carried out on a special table provided with a lead screen.

3. Proximity to the radium must be for as short a time as possible.

4. The time at which the radium treatment is begun and the time at which it is due to be terminated must be carefully noted. The success of the treatment and the safety of the patient depend on careful calculation of the dosage to be employed. The time during which the radium is in contact with the tissues is one factor in these calculations.

5. Careful checking of the radium is essential. The theatre nurse or sister is responsible for checking the containers when brought to the theatre and when removed from the sterilizer. The amount of radium, the

number and size of the needles used are entered on a
record card; unused containers are checked and returned to the radium safe.

Radium is a valuable substance and the careful
checking at each stage is the best safeguard against acci-
dental loss. Radium is also a dangerous substance.
Radium containers left about in the theatre or ward or a
radium needle that has slipped from its proper site and
is lying in contact with healthy tissue constitute a risk in
the one instance to the hospital personnel and in the
other instance to the patient.

It is usual to issue rules for the guidance of those concerned with the care of radium and the nursing of
patients undergoing radium treatment and a disc showing the radiation symbol is attached to the bed. In the
theatre a special card is filled in giving details of the
number and type of needles and containers used,
the time of insertion and of removal. This card is sent to
the ward when the patient leaves the theatre and is
completed when the radium is removed.

Radioactive Isotopes

Isotopes are variations of an element which have iden-
tical chemical properties but different atomic weights.
Most elements have at least two isotopes. The radioactive isotopes of certain elements which are now being
used in medical treatment are artificially produced by
the bombardment of the nuclei of the atoms in an atomic
pile. The radioactive isotopes used in medicine are in
fact by-products of the atomic research stations.

Examples of radioactive isotopes found to have a
medical use are:

Radioactive iodine in the treatment of thyrotoxicosis

E

and of carcinoma of the thyroid gland. A measured dose is given by mouth and absorbed into the blood stream from the alimentary tract. From the blood it is deposited in the thyroid gland and there acts as a source of localized radiation. The iodine is given in sufficient dosage to obliterate excessive thyroid tissue, or in the case of carcinoma, in patients over the age of forty-five years to destroy the malignant cells.

Radioactive phosphorus. This has been found effective in the treatment of polycythaemia, a condition in which the blood contains an excessive number of red cells. The phosphorus may be given by mouth or by intravenous injection.

Radioactive cobalt. This has a long 'life' compared with most other radioactive isotopes; it loses half its strength in rather more than 5 years. It is used in a beam unit and has an effect similar to that of high voltage X-ray therapy.

Radioactive gold. This is used locally in the peritoneal or pleural cavities in cases of malignant disease where secondary deposits cause large peritoneal or pleural effusions necessitating frequent aspiration. The use of gold for this purpose has proved successful in reducing the effusion and thereby saving the patient considerable discomfort. Radioactive gold is also introduced into the peritoneal cavity after operation for a malignant condition if there is a possibility of an 'overspill' of malignant cells, as, for example, from an ovarian cyst, or if minute deposits are known to be present in the peritoneum when the primary growth is removed.

Radioactive Tracers

Radioactive isotopes are useful assistants in solving

physiological and medical problems. Very minute quantities can be traced in the body by means of a delicate instrument, the Geiger counter. If, for example, radioactive iodine is used not for the treatment of disease of the thyroid gland, but to assess the activity of the gland, a small dose is given by mouth and the Geiger counter is set up in position over the thyroid area and will record the arrival of the radioactive isotope in the tissues of the gland. If there is no active thyroid tissue no iodine will be taken up; if there is enlargement and/or increased activity of the gland the absorption of the iodine will be more rapid than normal.

This ability to act as tracers in the body is providing one of the most useful fields for the employment of radioactive isotopes.

Precautions to be Taken

All persons working with radioactive substances or X-rays must observe the regulations laid down for their protection or their health will sooner or later be affected. Prolonged exposure to even small doses of radiation will damage the bone marrow and eventually diminish the supply of blood cells. The germ plasm of the ovaries and testes is damaged by radiation and sterility may result. In the early days of the use of X-rays repeated exposure of the hands caused destruction of the skin, ulceration and later malignant changes. All staff working in X-ray departments or with ionizing radiation carry monitoring film badges which record any exposure to radiation.

In the handling of radioactive isotopes similar precautions are required as in dealing with other forms of radiation, but in addition there is the danger of contamination with radioactive particles. If the worker's hands become contaminated there is danger of swallowing these particles. Radioactive dust may be inhaled during the course of the work. Therefore, in addition to working behind protective screens, protective clothing, including rubber gloves, is worn. Handling radioactive material is carried out by means of long-handled tools and instruments. It is of course essential that no eating, drinking or smoking should be allowed during such work.

When patients are receiving doses of radioactive iodine some of the material will be excreted in the urine, most of it within the first 48 hours. Typical regulations are quoted below.

Areas of treated skin may be washed with soap and water but must be thoroughly dried. Frequent non-irritating fluids to drink and mouth washes of glycerin and thymol will help. Mist. aspirin or mist. paracetamol will relieve soreness of mouth and throat and mist. lignocaine is used to rinse the mouth. Graneodin ointment may be used for external application. Palpation and washing of the neck by nurses should be avoided.

Patients are required to use one designated toilet which should be flushed twice after use and monitored periodically. When a bedpan or urinal is used, it should be emptied immediately and then washed and rinsed with sodium iodide with splashing avoided. Rubber gloves are worn.

Vomit. After emptying and washing bowls used in the first 24 hours, they should be placed in plastic bags and stored until monitoring is possible.

Faeces. No precautions are required.

Hands. To avoid contamination of the hands, rubber gloves are worn when attending to an incontinent patient receiving therapy doses. Gloves should be washed on the hands before they are removed. The hands must be washed after removing the gloves and again before eating or smoking.

In the case of small tracer doses of radioactive material these stringent precautions are not considered necessary. Contaminated equipment, clothing and bed linen should be handled with rubber gloves, placed in plastic bags and stored outside the ward until taken away by the staff of the Physics Department.

18. Food Requirements

The normal daily diet should contain proteins, carbohydrates and fats for energy, growth and repair, in the following proportions:

Protein, 10 to 15% of the whole.
Carbohydrate, 50 to 60% of the whole.
Fat, 30 to 35% of the whole.

In addition, the body needs water, vitamins and salts. These are usually present in sufficient quantities for health in the average mixed diet. Thirst is normally an adequate guide to fluid intake, but at least 2 litres (4 pints) per day are normally required, besides the water obtained from most foods and from oxidation of food in the body.

It is recommended that the protein in the daily diet should average 1 g per kg of body weight.

Calorie Requirements

The energy requirements of the body are measured in units of heat or calories. The Calorie (or kilocalorie) as used in dietetic calculations represents the amount of heat needed to raise 1 kilogram of water (1 litre) through 1° C.

Basal Metabolic Requirements

These represent the minimum energy requirements for sustaining bodily functions such as respiration and heart action during complete physical rest or sleep. More than half the Calories obtained from the daily food intake are required for basal metabolism, i.e. about 1,800 for an average healthy man and about 1,500 for an average healthy woman. Tables are available so that for any person whose height, weight, age and sex are known, the energy value of total food intake can be calculated with reasonable accuracy.

Average Daily Calorie Requirements

	Men 70 kg	Women 56 kg
Weight:		
Sedentary (36 Cal. per kg)	2,500	2,000
Moderately active (43 Cal. per kg)	3,000	2,400
Very active (64 Cal. per kg)	4,000 or more	3,000

Age last birthday (years)	Boys	Girls
1	1,050	1,050
3	1,470	1,470
5	1,800	1,800
6	1,950	1,920
10	2,420	2,250
14	3,000	2,350
15	3,300	2,550
18	3,300	2,550

Pregnancy and Lactation

During the latter half of pregnancy and during lactation the mother's diet needs to be adequate but not excessive. A daily intake producing 2,500 to 3,000 Calories may be regarded as average requirements. The protein proportion should be increased to 1·5 g per kg of body weight.

Additional requirements are:

iron 15 to 20 mg
vitamin A, 6,000 I.U. } International Units
vitamin D, 600 I.U.

Dietary Requirements in Illness

The factors which alter the body's requirements during illness should influence the choice of diet for the patient. Because he is lying inactive in bed his Calorie requirements will not necessarily be small. For example, trauma to body tissues as a result of burns, accidents, surgery or infection will result in excessive protein loss and the nurse must see that protein in excess of normal requirements is supplied. The permeability of blood capillaries may be affected if Vitamin C is short in the diet and as a good blood supply is a prerequisite of healing tissue, this must also be included in sufficient quantities. At the time of admission, or subsequently, a patient's emotional state may inhibit the secretion of gastric juice, so affecting his digestion. He should be reassured and helped to feel relaxed and self confident. Presentation, size of helping and digestibility of the food offered may restore his appetite.

A knowledge of Calorie requirements alone is insufficient. The diet should be balanced to include the essential nutrients in the right proportion to each other and to the metabolic needs of the patient. Carbohydrates may supply sufficient Calories but will not meet the nutritional needs of a growing boy or a patient who requires extra protein and Vitamin C. Tables are available showing the amounts of the different nutrients needed, in health and in illness, for example:

> 1 g of Protein gives roughly 4 Calories.
> 1 g of Carbohydrate gives roughly 4 Calories.
> 1 g of Fat gives roughly 9 Calories.

Tables are also available stating either the percentage or weight of carbohydrate, protein and fats in relation to the needs of the patient.

Dietetics is the science of regulating diet. In hospital this can be applied successfully in relation to particular organs affected by disease, e.g. the carbohydrate intake is regulated in the treatment of diabetes mellitus. Most hospitals have a trained dietician and a special kitchen where the many different diets are prepared.

Some diets may be unpopular with the patient, e.g. the reducing diet. The nurse can do much to help the patient accept his diet by explaining its function in meeting his particular needs and by seeing that it is served promptly and attractively. The nurse must be prepared to offer an alternative of equivalent dietary value if a patient cannot accept a specific item of food on religious grounds.

A knowledge of nutrition equips the nurse, as a health teacher, to help her patients with various problems associated not only with diet in disease but good diet as a means of preventing illness.

When the diet is supplied in fluid form, for example to the unconscious patient, proprietary foods are available containing the essential nutrients in a concentrated form. These can be administered through a Ryle's tube. Where intragastric feeding is not possible, sterile solutions of concentrated nutrients are available for intravenous administration. (See p. 40.)

Proprietary Foods

Name	Contents	Analysis
Aminolipid vitrum for tube feeding	Casein hydrolysate	8 g
	Arachis oil	36·5 g
	Glucose	10·0 g

Name	*Contents*	*Analysis*
Aminolipid vitrum (*cont.*)	Emulsifying agents	
	Water to	100 ml contains 400 Cal./100 ml

Note: Because of the high fat content it is advisable not to give more than 300 ml daily.

Casilan	Contains	protein	90%
		fat	1·8%
		Na⁺less than	0·1%
		Ca⁺⁺	1·2%
Complan	Contains	protein	31%
		fat	16%
		carbohydrate	44%
		Ca⁺⁺	0·8%
		Na⁺	0·4%
		K⁺	1·1%

Note: Also contains vitamins and iron and is a complete food suitable for intragastric tube-feeding when dissolved in water.

100 g yields 450 Calories

Intragastric feeds of Complan and Casilan tend to produce diarrhoea in some patients, and the feed may need to be diluted at first. It should not be given in a concentration greater than 15%.

Edosol	A low sodium milk powder	
	contains protein	28%
	carbohydrate	36·5%
	fat	28%
	sodium less than	0·03%

1 oz yields 150 Calories
100 g yields 520 Calories

Name	*Contents*
Prosparol	Contains arachis oil in 50% emulsion in water, and yields 450 Cal./100 ml. Contains no carbohydrate or fat. May be given orally with flavourings and fruit juices, or by intragastric drip. The daily intake should not exceed 300 ml.

VITAMIN CHART

Vitamin	Properties and Deficiency Effects*
A Fat soluble. Slowly destroyed by exposure to air or light. Rapidly destroyed by rancidity of fat.	Necessary for health and growth, for maintaining healthy mucous membranes and skin and for the normal functioning of the visual purple in the eye. *Deficiency Effects* *Mild:* Lowered resistance to infection, night blindness. *Severe:* Xerophthalmia, infection of mucous membrane.
B complex All water soluble.	
B_1 Aneurin. Anti neuritic.	Concerned with cell respiration and carbohydrate metabolism. *Deficiency Effects* *Mild:* Loss of appetite, digestive disturbances, debility, retarded growth, nervous disorders, insomnia. *Severe:* Beri-beri, polyneuritis, paralysis.
B_2 Riboflavine. Less stable when exposed to light.	Like B_1, it forms a link in the chain of processes through which the body obtains energy from carbohydrates and is necessary for healthy skin. *Deficiency Effects* *Mild:* Digestive disturbances, burning and soreness of the eyes, lips and tongue, weakness, retarded growth. *Severe:* Diarrhoea, dermatitis, loss of hair, sores at the angle of the mouth, corneal opacities.

* *Note:* Vitamins are regarded as essential for growth and health, although it is difficult to define accurately the part played by some of them in normal development and in the maintenance of health.

Good Natural Sources	*Optimum Daily Requirements*
Fish, liver oils, most meats, butter, cheese, oily fish, margarine, green vegetables, carrots, tomatoes, apricots.	Infants to Adolescents: 1,000 to 5,000 I.U. Adults: 3,000 I.U. Pregnancy and Lactation: 6,000 to 8,000 I.U.
Almost all foods except white flour and sugar.	About 1·5 mg to 2 mg
Milk, eggs, cheese, liver, kidney, yeast, wholemeal bread.	Children: 1·5 mg Adults: 1·5 mg to 2 mg

Vitamin	Properties and Deficiency Effects
B₆ Pyridoxine. Unstable to light.	Concerned with protein metabolism and healthy skin.
B₁₂ Cyanocobalamin. Anti-pernicious anaemia factor. See p. 91.	
Others in the B complex group: Nicotinic Acid Anti pellagra	Function similar to that of Riboflavine. *Deficiency Effects* *Mild:* Loss of weight, sore tongue, mouth infections, rough red skin, especially parts exposed to light. *Severe:* Pellagra (symptoms: diarrhoea, dermatitis, dementia).
Pantothenic Acid. Biotin. Folic acid.	Health of skin. Similar to Vitamin B₁₂ used in the treatment of macrocytic anaemia.
C Ascorbic acid. Water soluble. Unstable to heat, but rapid cooking less destructive than long slow cooking. No destruction in modern canning of fruit and vegetables.	Necessary for production of normal endothelial and epithelial cells and for growth. *Deficiency Effects* *Mild:* Slow healing of wounds and fractures, anaemia, infection of mouth and gums. *Severe:* Scurvy (tender swollen extremities, subcutaneous and submucous haemorrhages).
D Calciferol. Anti-rachitic. Fat soluble.	Regulates metabolism of calcium and phosphorus, necessary for growth of bones and teeth. *Deficiency Effects* *Mild:* Poor muscle tone, retarded skeletal growth. *Severe:* Rickets, osteomalacia.

Good Natural Sources	*Optimum Daily Requirements*
Unpolished rice or rice bran, whole cereals, yeast, milk, liver, wheat germ, small amounts in most foods.	10 to 20 mg
Meat, whole cereals, yeast, bacon.	10 to 20 mg (N.B. May cause vaso-dilation)
Fresh fruit and vegetables, blackcurrant juice either fresh or sold in bottles bearing on the label the amount of Vit. C present.	30 mg to 50 mg
Fish-liver oils, eggs, butter, margarine. Vitamin D can also be produced in the body by exposure to sunlight or ultra violet light.	Infants, pregnant and lactating women: 600 to 800 I.U. Children: 400 I.U. Adults: 200 I.U.

Vitamin	*Properties and Deficiency Effects*
E Fat soluble.	The properties of this particular vitamin are therapeutically as yet, uncertain, although it may be used to produce peripheral vaso-dilation.
K Anti-haemorrhagic. Fat soluble.	Essential for maintaining the normal blood-clotting function. Bile is necessary for the absorption of vitamin K. *Deficiency Effects* Prolonged bleeding and clotting times. Often associated with obstructive jaundice and diseases of the liver.

Most modern diets contain adequate vitamins and only the young, the aged or the pregnant woman are likely to need vitamin supplements. Sufficient vitamins should be given to improve the patient's condition only to a point where a normal diet will supply all the necessary nutrients.

Good Natural Sources	Optimum Daily Requirements
Wheat germ oil, oats, milk, green leaves and lettuce.	
Deficiency unlikely if person is eating a well balanced diet.	

Vitamins can also be given therapeutically in the form of tablets or capsules for oral administration or by injection, e.g. Vitamin A capsules or ABIDEC containing vitamins A B$_1$ B$_2$ B$_6$ C and D and Nicotinamide. Vitamin K may be given prophylactically to persons undergoing surgery and who have a tendency to bleed excessively or to patients having anticoagulant drugs if they should start to bleed.

MINERAL INORGANIC ELEMENTS

The main requirements are calcium, copper, iodine, iron, phosphorus, potassium and sodium.

Name	Biological properties	Good natural sources
Calcium	Necessary for all body processes, particularly bone and teeth formation during years of growth. An essential constituent of blood. *Daily needs:* in pregnancy 1·5 g; childhood/adolescence 1 to 1·4 g; for adults 1 g	Milk, milk products, especially cheese, dried milk; egg yolk, green leafy vegetables, especially outer leaves, oats, rice, wheat, legumes, nuts, coconut, citrus fruits, dried figs, lettuce, carrots, sardines.
Copper	Speeds up formation of haemoglobin of red blood cells. Very minute amount needed.	Sufficient amounts present in any well-balanced diet.
Iodine	Minute amounts needed by thyroid gland in making thyroxin.	Water, fish, vegetables. Iodized table salt can supplement natural sources.
Iron	Essential constituent of haemoglobin in red blood cells. Average daily need: 10 to 15 mg.	Meat, liver, kidneys, egg yolk, fish, especially saltwater fish, oat meal, black treacle, maize, rice, wheat, legumes, nuts, coconut, dried figs, carrots, green and yellow vegetables and fruits. In apples, peaches and apricots the iron lies just under the skin.
Phosphorus	Needed for normal functioning of cells; for bones and teeth, calcium phosphate being the chief inorganic constituent of bone. Amount contained in a mixed diet is ample.	Meat, fish, liver, brains, pancreas, etc., milk, dried milk, cheese, egg yolk, barley, kaffir-corn, maize, millet, oats, rice, wheat, legumes, nuts, coconut, plums, dried figs, lettuce, carrots, cocoa.

Name	Biological properties	Good natural sources
Potassium	Essential constituent of the body cells.	Present in many substances in a normal diet.
Sodium	A constituent of body cells and fluids. Is most abundant in the extracellular fluid. 5 g daily should be ample. More salt is needed in hot climates where loss of water and salt through sweating is usual.	Sodium (sodium chloride) is the only salt eaten as such. Found in all animal cells e.g. meat, and present in most foods as part of their chemical make-up.

19. Metric—Imperial Conversion Tables

The metric system of weights and measures is replacing the traditional imperial system in Britain. The metric system is international, it is a simpler and therefore safer system to use in calculating drug dosages. A knowledge of both systems will be needed for reference for some time, however, since the transition is not yet completed everywhere.

FLUID MEASURES (approximate*)

Millilitres	Minims	Millilitres	Minims
10	150	0·8	12
8	120	0·6	10
6	90	0·5	8
5	75	0·4	6
4	60	0·3	5
3	45	0·25	4
2·6	40	0·2	3
2	30	0·15	2½
1·6	25	0·12	2
1·3	20	0·1	1½
1	15	0·06	1

1 fluid ounce	= approx. 30 ml
1 fluid drachm	= approx. 4 ml
15 minims	= approx. 1 ml

* *N.B.—These approximations may be used for the direct transference of doses from one system to the other. Multiples of these equivalents must not be used since, in multiplying, the error of the approximation might be raised to a significant figure (see Table of accurate equivalents).*

DOSAGE WEIGHTS (approximate*)

Grams	Grains		Milligrams	Grains
10	150		40	$\frac{2}{3}$
8	120		30	$\frac{1}{2}$
6	90		25	$\frac{2}{5}$
5	75		20	$\frac{1}{3}$
4	60		16	$\frac{1}{4}$
3	45		12	$\frac{1}{5}$
2·6	40		10	$\frac{1}{6}$
2	30		8	$\frac{1}{8}$
1·6	25		6	$\frac{1}{10}$
1·3	20		5	$\frac{1}{12}$
1	15		4	$\frac{1}{16}$
0·8	12		3	$\frac{1}{20}$
0·6	10		2·5	$\frac{1}{24}$
0·5	8		2	$\frac{1}{30}$
			1·5	$\frac{1}{40}$
Milligrams	Grains		1·2	$\frac{1}{50}$
400	6		1	$\frac{1}{60}$
300	5		0·8	$\frac{1}{80}$
250	4		0·6	$\frac{1}{100}$
200	3		0·5	$\frac{1}{120}$
150	$2\frac{1}{2}$		0·4	$\frac{1}{160}$
120	2		0·3	$\frac{1}{200}$
100	$1\frac{1}{2}$		0·25	$\frac{1}{240}$
80	$1\frac{1}{3}$		0·2	$\frac{1}{320}$
75	$1\frac{1}{4}$		0·15	$\frac{1}{400}$
60	1		0·12	$\frac{1}{500}$
50	$\frac{3}{4}$		0·1	$\frac{1}{600}$

* See note on opposite page.

BODY WEIGHT (approximate*)

Grams (g)	Ounces (oz)	Grams (g)	Ounces (oz)
30	1·0	250	8·7
50	1·7	275	9·6
75	2·6	300	10·5
100	3·5	325	11·4
125	4·4	350	12·2
150	5·2	375	13·1
175	6·1	400	14·0
200	7·0	425	14·9
225	7·9		

Kilograms (kg)	Pounds (lb)	Kilograms (kg)	Pounds (lb)
0·5	1 lb 2 oz	3·5	7 lb 14 oz
1·0	2 lb 4 oz	4·0	9 lb
1·5	3 lb 6 oz	4·5	10 lb 2 oz
2·0	4 lb 8 oz	5·0	11 lb 4 oz
2·5	5 lb 10 oz	5·5	12 lb 6 oz
3·0	6 lb 12 oz	6·0	13 lb 8 oz

Kilograms (kg)	Stone (st)	Kilograms (kg)	Stone (st)
8	1 st 4 lb	55	8 st 12 lb
10	1 st 8 lb	60	9 st 9 lb
15	2 st 6 lb	65	10 st 6 lb
20	3 st 3 lb	70	11 st 3 lb
25	4 st	75	12 st
30	4 st 11 lb	80	12 st 11 lb
35	5 st 9 lb	85	13 st 9 lb
40	6 st 6 lb	90	14 st 6 lb
45	7 st 3 lb	95	15 st 3 lb
50	8 st	100	16 st

* See note on p. 130.

ACCURATE CONVERSION FACTORS

N.B.—The following precise equivalents should always be used for multiple conversion factors.

Weight or Mass

1 kilogram (kg)	= 15,432 grains
	or 35·274 ounces
	or 2·2046 pounds
1 gram (g or G)	= 15·432 grains
1 milligram (mg)	= 0·015432 grain
1 microgram (μg)	= 0·000015 grain
1 pound (avoirdupois) (lb)	= 453·59 grams
1 ounce (avoirdupois) (oz)	= 28·35 grams
1 grain (gr)	= 64·799 milligrams

Fluid Volume or Capacity

1 litre (1)	= 1·7598 pints
	or 0·22 gallons
1 millilitre (ml)	= 16·894 minims
1 litre (1)	= 0·0353 cubic feet
1 pint	= 568·25 millilitres
	or 0·56825 litres
1 fluid ounce (fl oz)	= 28·412 millilitres
1 fluid drachm (fl dr)	= 3·5515 millilitres
1 minim (m or min)	= 0·059192 millilitres

Length

1 metre (m)	= 39·370 inches
1 decimetre (dm)	= 3·9370 inches
1 centimetre (cm)	= 0·3937 inches
1 millimetre (mm)	= 0·03937 inches

1 inch	= 25·400 millimetres
1 foot	= 30·48 centimetres
1 yard	= 0·914 metres

Other Measures in Common Use

The nurse may need to know the following measures:
1 mega unit (e.g. for penicillin) = 1,000,000 units
1 ml = 16 minims = 15 or 16 drops.

Approximate Domestic Measurements

The plastic teaspoon manufactured specifically for use in the administration of medicines holds 5 ml.

1 average sized tumbler holds *approx.*			200 ml
1 teacup	„	„	150 ml
1 soup plate (half-full)	„	„	200 ml
1 glass jug (when full to the top)	„	„	1 litre
1 dessert spoon full	„	„	10 ml

N.B. These measures must obviously not be used for measuring drugs.

Method of Calculating a Dosage

Dosages administered in the metric system are usually straightforward, requiring only a simple division or multiplication, but occasionally a more difficult dosage is prescribed.

Example: The ampoule of the drug contains 250 mg in 2 ml. The dose prescribed is 100 mg.

$$250 \text{ mg are contained in } 2 \text{ ml}$$

$$\therefore \quad 100 \text{ mg are contained in } \frac{100 \times 2}{250} \text{ ml}$$

$$= \tfrac{4}{5}\text{th ml}$$

Note: For examples involving decimal points see p. 137.

Percentage Solutions

'Percentage' is used to denote the strength of a solution, which may be a weight in volume (W/V) or a volume in volume (V/V) solution.

W/V solution means that the solute is a solid which must be measured in weight, whereas the solvent is a liquid and must be measured in volume units.

V/V solution means that both the solute and the solvent are liquids and therefore both are measured in volume units.

A volume % may also be a measurement of the amount of gas dissolved in a liquid. For example, when 10 ml of gas is dissolved in 100 ml of fluid, the concentration can be expressed as 10 volumes %.

1 % solution prepared according to the metric system is equivalent to 1 g in 100 ml and prepared according to the Apothecaries' System is equivalent to 1 grain in 110 minims.

Dilution of Lotions

Where instructions are not supplied regarding the dilutions required, the following formula can be used:

$$\frac{\text{Strength required}}{\text{Strength of Stock Solution}} \times \text{ Volume required}$$

This formula may be abbreviated to:

$$\frac{\text{Want}}{\text{Have}} \times \text{ Amount}$$

Example: To prepare 600 ml of 1 in 30 solution from a
            stock solution of 1 in 10.

$$\frac{\frac{1}{30} \text{ (strength reqd.)}}{\frac{1}{10} \text{ (stock soltn.)}} \times 600 \text{ (vol. reqd.)} \quad \text{ml stock soltn.}$$

Note. To divide by a fraction, e.g. $\frac{1}{10}$, turn it 'upside
         down' and multiply, viz. $\frac{10}{1}$

$$\frac{1}{30} \times \frac{10}{1} \times 600 \text{ ml stock solution}$$

$$= 200 \text{ ml stock solution}$$

As 600 ml of 1 in 30 solution is required, 400 ml of water
must be added to the 200 ml stock solution to produce
600 ml at a dilution of 1 in 30.

To dilute a stock solution of known percentage to a
weaker solution, use the same formula.

Note. To express a ratio as a %, multiply by 100

Example: 1 in 20

$$= \tfrac{1}{20} \times 100 = 5\%$$

To express a % as a ratio, divide by 100

Example: 20%

$$= \frac{100}{20} = 5 = 1 \text{ in } 5.$$

If the problem includes both a ratio and a percentage,
convert one to the other.

Example: To prepare 400 ml of 0·02% solution from a stock solution of 1 in 200 solution.

$$\frac{\text{% of strength required}}{\text{% of stock soltn.}} \times \text{volume required}$$

Thus:

$$\frac{0·02}{0·5 \text{ (i.e. } \frac{1}{200} \times 100)} \times 400 \text{ ml}$$

= 16 ml stock solution.

400 — 16 = 384 ml
16 ml stock soltn. + 384 ml water
= 400 ml 0·02 solution.

Note. Some nurses might find it easier to eliminate the decimal point completely as in the same example:

$$\frac{2}{50} \times 400 \text{ ml} = 16 \text{ ml}$$

In the first fraction the decimal point has been moved two places to the right, therefore two 0's have been added to the 100.

Similarly the second fraction has the decimal point moved one place and therefore one 0 has to be added to the 100.

20. Thermometric Conversion Scales

*N.B.—The following tables are approximate and may be
used for direct transference from one system to the other.
For accurate conversion factors, to be used in multiples,
see below.*

Centigrade (°C)	Fahrenheit (°F)	Centigrade (°C)	Fahrenheit (°F)
110	230	38	100·4
100—Boiling point—**212**		37·5	99·5
of water			
95	203	37	98·6
90	194	36·5	97·7
85	185	36	96·8
80	176	35·5	95·9
75	167	35	95·0
70	158	34	93·2
65	149	33	91·4
60	140	32	89·6
55	131	31	87·6
50	122	30	86
45	113	25	77
44	111·2	20	68
43	109·4	15	59
42	107·6	10	50
41	105·8	5	41
40·5	104·9	**0**—Freezing point—**32**	
		of water	
40	104·0	— 5	23
39·5	103·1	—10	14
39	102·2	—15	5
38·5	101·3	—20	—4

To convert Fahrenheit into Centigrade, subtract 32, multiply the remainder by 5, and divide the result by 9. To convert Centigrade to Fahrenheit, multiply by 9, divide by 5, and add 32.

$0°$ C ($32°F$) = temperature of melting ice at sea level.
$100°$ C ($212°F$) = temperature of steam given off when water is boiled under atmospheric pressure at sea level.

Thermometers

Clinical. In normal use this has a scale between $35°$ and $43°$ C or $95°$ to $110°F$.

Rectal. This is similar, but is usually distinguished by a blue-coloured bulb.

Low reading. This has a scale of $25°$ to $40°$ C and is used when temperatures below the normal scales are suspected, e.g. where elderly people are admitted in winter with suspected hypothermia or sometimes in cases of hypothyroidism.

Induced hypothermia. Special thermometers are used which can pass into the naso-pharynx, oesophagus, trachea, rectum, skin or muscle. Those used are connected by leads to an electric recording machine for a continuous recording.

Temperatures

For irrigations. Lotions for swabbing wounds and irrigating body cavities should be used at $38°$ C ($100·4°F$) unless there are orders to the contrary.

Syringing the external auditory meatus with lotion that is materially hotter or colder than the body temperature will stimulate the semicircular canals of the internal ear and may cause giddiness and nausea.

Baby bath. The temperature of the water should be 38° C (100·4°F).

Tepid sponging. The temperature of the water is usually about 30° C at the commencement and this is gradually reduced to roughly 24° C (86° to 75·2°F). If very cold sponging is ordered, the water used should be kept as near 0° C as possible by the addition of ice.

21. The Examination of Urine

Collection of Specimens of Urine

Usually a specimen of the urine passed on waking in the early morning is required for routine testing; if a patient is admitted to hospital as an urgent case, a specimen of urine should be obtained as soon as possible. The first morning specimen of urine passed by a diabetic patient should be discarded, as urine which has been accumulating in the bladder during the night does not give an accurate result. Specimens should be collected into clean, dry containers; contact with disinfectants or detergents can affect the results of some chemical tests. Whether in the ward or in the laboratory, testing should be carried out with freshly passed urine; if the specimen has been left to stand and decomposition has begun, important constituents may be altered or destroyed.

Specimens for Bacteriological Examination

These specimens are collected into sterile urine containers and aseptic precautions are observed. In the case of a woman patient a catheter specimen may be required. Catheterization, however careful the aseptic technique may be, carries some risk of infection and a 'clean' specimen of urine may be considered suitable for both male and female patients.

To Collect a 'Clean' Specimen of Urine

The external genital organs are first thoroughly washed with soap and water. The area around the urethral orifice is swabbed with a suitable mildly antiseptic lotion.

The patient is then asked to micturate, and when a small quantity of urine has been passed a mid-stream specimen is collected in a sterile jar.

The specimen is labelled and sent to the laboratory immediately.

To collect a 24-hour specimen of urine (e.g. from 8 a.m. one day to 8 a.m. the following day):

8 a.m. The patient is asked to empty his bladder and the urine is discarded. Every time the patient passes urine throughout the ensuing 24 hours, the whole amount passed is saved in a large container.

8 a.m. At the end of the 24-hour period the patient is asked to empty his bladder and this urine is added to that already in the collecting jar.

For examination for the presence of *Mycobacterium tuberculosis* a specimen of the urine containing some of the sediment from the bottom of the jar is required.

A 24-hour specimen may be required for chemical examination and in this case the entire amount collected is usually sent to the laboratory.

Observation of Volume, Colour, Deposits, Specific Gravity and Reaction Volume

An adult in health excretes about 1 to 1·5 litres of urine in 24 hours, but this can vary considerably, being influenced by the fluid intake and by loss of fluid by other routes such as, for example, variations in the amount of water lost through the skin as sweat.

In some diseases the urinary output increases; for example in chronic renal failure when the kidney is unable to concentrate the urine, diabetes mellitus where the amount of urine increases in order to dilute and excrete glucose, which is not normally present in the urine, and diabetes insipidus, a condition in which the pituitary gland fails to produce the water-retaining (anti-diuretic) hormone. Decrease in the urinary output (oliguria) occurs in nephritis, acute renal failure, any condition which reduces the blood supply to the kidneys, circulatory failure from any cause, cardiac failure. Toxic chemicals also produce oliguria by damaging the kidney—e.g. sulphonamides, arsenical compounds, mercury. *Accurate* measurement of the volume of urine passed is essential in many pathological conditions.

Colour. Urine is usually described as pale amber, but the colour varies according to the concentration of the urine in the particular specimen observed. Very dilute urine is almost colourless, while concentrated urine is dark yellow. The colour is altered by the presence of some abnormal constituents. A significant amount of blood will colour the urine red or a smoky-brown, bile gives it a greenish-brown colour. Dyes excreted in the urine can also alter the colour as, for example, the blue urine seen after the administration of indigo-carmine or 'Diagnex' Azure A exchange resin. Blackcurrant juice or beetroot, taken in sufficient quantities will colour the urine red.

Deposits. When urine is collected in a specimen glass and allowed to stand a deposit can usually be seen which is due to the precipitation of normal urinary constituents, urates and phosphates.

Mucus, pus, red blood cells and epithelial casts from the renal tubules are some abnormal substances which may form a deposit, which in such cases is usually required for microscopic examination.

Specific gravity. The specific gravity of a substance is the weight of 1 litre of that substance compared with the weight of 1 litre of distilled water, which is 1000 grammes.

The specific gravity of normal urine ranges from 1003 to 1030, varying with the fluid intake and fluid loss which will affect the concentration of the urine. A high specific gravity with a large volume of urine is found in diabetes mellitus, due to the presence of sugar.

A persistently low specific gravity is one of the signs of renal failure. (See renal function tests, pp. 168, 169.)

Specific gravity of urine is measured with a glass instrument known as a urinometer. There must be a sufficient quantity of urine in the specimen glass to enable the urinometer to float in the fluid without touching the bottom of the glass. The figure read on the stem of the urinometer at the level of the surface of the urine gives the specific gravity.

If the volume of the sample of urine obtained is insufficient to float the urinometer, then the sample may be sent to the laboratory where other methods of estimating the specific gravity can be used.

Reaction. Normal urine is usually slightly acid, although urine passed immediately after a meal may be alkaline. If a specimen of urine is left to stand it will become alkaline owing to the conversion of urea into ammonia.

Litmus paper is commonly used to test the reaction of a specimen of urine. Acid urine turns blue litmus paper red. Alkaline urine turns red litmus paper blue. Neutral urine does not alter the colour of either red or blue litmus.

Abnormal Constituents which may be present in Urine
Protein. Plasma proteins do not normally pass from the blood to the urine, but may do so when the renal tubules

are damaged; for example in acute nephritis, the nephro-tic syndrome, and damage due to toxins. Proteinuria (albuminuria) may also be present in acute febrile con-ditions and in congestive cardiac failure. Occasionally it occurs in healthy young adults; protein appears in the urine at the end of the day, but after a night's rest it disappears. This condition, which is known as 'postural proteinuria', is not usually associated with any disease process and clears up spontaneously.

Glucose. The presence of glucose in the urine is usually an indication of diabetes mellitus, but is occasionally due to other hormone disturbances or to a non-pathological condition where the renal-threshold for glucose is lower than normal and as a result the kidneys may excrete some glucose following the intake of a considerable quantity of carbohydrate.

Acetone and diacetic acid. These ketone bodies are formed and excreted as a result of the incomplete meta-bolism of fats associated with some abnormality of car-bohydrate metabolism.

In diabetes mellitus the presence of acetone and diace-tic acid in the urine is a warning of the possibility of diabetic coma.

Blood. Blood may be found in the urine of patients suffering from disease or injury of the urinary tract; as, for example, acute nephritis, renal or vesical stones, new growths, bilharzial infestation, tuberculosis of the kid-ney, or crush injuries involving the kidney or bladder.

Bile. Bile is present in the urine in cases of obstructive jaundice, for example a gall-stone in the common bile duct, and in inflammatory diseases of the liver, such as infective hepatitis.

Pus. Pus may be found in the urine in any infection of the urinary tract, cystitis, pyelitis, associated with renal calculi and also in tuberculous infection.

Testing Urine

It is now common practice for proprietary strips and tablet reagents to be used for testing urine by showing colour changes. Some of these demonstrate the presence of abnormal constituents whilst others indicate the quantity. Strips impregnated with several reagents permit several tests to be made simultaneously.

Clear instructions and colour charts are issued in the use of these different tests. If they are not followed meticulously with regard to the number of drops of urine and/or water to be used and the exact timing for observations, inaccuracies may result. A standardized test tube and dropper must also be used in conjunction with these products and filter paper must not be substituted for the test mats as the texture is incorrect. When a colour comparison is to be made, it is important that the colour chart is held close enough to the test. It is not necessary, when using these particular tests, to filter the urine or to acidify it but one must still avoid testing stale alkaline urine.

It is customary in out-patient clinics and on first admitting a patient to test first for the presence of abnormalities and then where abnormalities are detected, to follow on with quantitative tests, before reporting the result to the doctor.

Routine Screening Test

1. *Using multiple strips*

Bili-labstix   Test for pH, protein, glucose, ketones bilirubin and blood.

Labstix	Test for pH, protein, glucose, ketones and blood.
Hema-combistix	Test for pH, protein, glucose and blood.
Uristix	Test for protein and glucose.

2. *Using single strips*

pH	Litmus paper or pH indicator.
Albumin	Albustix.
Glucose	Clinistix (Specific for glucose, more sensitive than Clinitest).
Ketones	Ketostix or Acetest.
Bilirubin	Ictotest or Ictostix.
Blood	Hemastix.

Diabetic Tests

Clinitest. Copper reduction test, sensitive to all reducing sugars, e.g. lactose, fructose and demonstrating a quantity of 0 to 2%.

Hepato/Biliary Tests

| Urobilistix | Test for urobilinogen. |
| Ictostix or Ictotest | Test for bilirubin. |

Phenylketone Tests or P.A.S. (para-amino salicyclic acid) in Urine

Phenistix. The instructions issued with these strips should be observed carefully as positive results may be masked when certain drugs have been administered. Although this is unlikely with babies, the tests may be used for adults in a mental hospital.

Quantitative Estimation for Protein

In some hospitals this test is performed in the laboratory,

when the result will be more accurate. Alternatively the nurse carries out the 'Esbach's test'. Most doctors prefer the urine to be diluted with water if the specific gravity is over 1008. The final reading must then be multiplied by the degree of dilution, e.g. if 60 ml water is added to 60 ml of urine the answer will be multiplied by 2. The urine should be filtered, if cloudy, and acidified with a few drops of acetic acid if it is alkaline. The albumino-meter is filled with urine to the letter marked 'U'. Esbach's reagent is then added as far as the letter 'R'. The cork is replaced and the tube gently shaken. It is then placed in the stand, labelled and the result recorded 24 hours later. The height of the precipitate represents the number of grams of albumin per litre of urine. Dividing this figure by 10 gives the percentage.

22. Laboratory Investigations

Laboratory investigations play a large part in modern medicine. They vary greatly in their complexity and significance, but most of them depend for their success not only upon the laboratory work but also upon the care and accuracy with which the specimens are collected and transmitted to the laboratory. It is therefore useful for the nurse to have some knowledge of the nature and purpose of these tests.

The Collection of Samples

All specimens sent to the laboratory should be as fresh as possible, for in many cases even a few hours' delay will render the specimen unsuitable for examination, due to bacterial decomposition or other causes.

All specimens must be clearly labelled to prevent loss.

Specimens should if possible be collected first thing in the morning before breakfast, because the taking of a meal may materially affect the level of some substances in the blood or urine. Taking and delivering the specimens early is also helpful to the laboratory staff in organizing their work load.

Specimens of Blood

When sending blood for examination the greatest care must be taken to avoid haemolysis of the specimen, for haemolysis almost invariably renders it unusable.

To avoid haemolysis the syringe and needle used must be dry, so sterilizing by dry heat in a hot air or infra-red oven is recommended when non-disposable syringes are used.

For some tests blood serum is required, whilst for others whole unclotted blood must be sent. To prevent clotting potassium oxalate or sodium citrate is added to the specimen. Usually the laboratory supplies tubes with the required quantity of potassium oxalate crystals already added.

Blood Specimens for Clinical Pathology

Blood Test	*Amount and Type of Blood Required*
Absolute indices	2·5 ml sequestrene
Acid phosphatase	5 ml clotted
Alcohol	2·5 ml clotted or sequestrene
Alkali reserve	*5 ml
Alkaline phosphatase	5 ml clotted
Amylase	5 ml clotted
Antibody (antenatal test)	8 to 10 ml clotted
Antistreptolysin titre	10 ml clotted
Barbiturates	10 ml heparinized
Berger Kahn (Kahn)	8 to 10 ml clotted
Bilirubin	5 to 10 ml clotted (see note re Rh. babies)
Blood count	2 to 3 ml sequestrene
Bromide	10 ml clotted
Bromsulphthalein	10 ml clotted (see also p. 165)
Brucella agglutination	5 to 10 ml clotted
C. reactive protein	3 to 5 ml clotted
Calcium	5 ml clotted
Chloride	5 ml heparinized
Cholesterol	5 ml oxalated
Cold agglutinins	5 ml clotted (to be sent to laboratory within 15 minutes of collection)
Coombs	5 ml clotted
Electrolytes	5 ml heparinized (for bicarbonate estimation—5 ml heparinized under oil)
Erythrocyte sedimentation rate	2 to 3 ml sequestrene
Fibrinogen	2·5 ml sequestrene
Folic acid	15–20 ml clotted
Gonococcal complement	
Fixation	*5–10 ml

*denotes that a special container must be obtained from the laboratory for this specimen.

Blood Test	Amount and Type of Blood Required
Grouping and cross matching	2–5 ml sequestrene and 10 ml clotted
Haematocrit	2·5 ml sequestrene
Kahn (see Berger Kahn)	
Lactic dehydrogenese (L.D.H.)	5 ml clotted
Lipase	10 ml clotted
Paul Bunnell	5 ml clotted
Potassium	*5 ml
Protein bound iron	*10 ml
Proteins	5 ml clotted
Prothrombin	*2 to 5 ml
Pyruvic acid	*10 ml
R.A. latex agglutination	3 to 5 ml clotted
Salicylate	5 ml clotted
S.G.O.T. and S.G.P.T. (serum transaminases)	5 ml clotted
Sodium	*5 ml
Thyocyanate	7 ml clotted
Thymol turbidity	2 ml clotted
Thyroid antibody	5 ml clotted
Toxoplasma dye	10 ml clotted
Treponema immobilization (T.P.I.)	*10 ml
Van der Bergh	5 ml clotted
Viral and rickettsial viruses	10 ml clotted. 2 specimens, 2nd 10–14 days after 1st
Vitami B$_{12}$ (serum)	15 to 20 ml clotted
Wasserman reaction	*10 ml
Urea	2·5 ml sequestrene
Uric acid	5 ml clotted

*denotes that a special container must be obtained from the laboratory for this specimen.

Hospital laboratories may differ over the type of container used and the type and amount of blood required for some of the tests. In cases of doubt the nurse should ask either the doctor who will be taking the blood or one of the laboratory staff.

A number of tests are carried out by laboratory staff who usually bring their own equipment with them; these differ from one hospital to another. Tests often performed by laboratory staff are:

Astrup (this may also   Haemaglobin
  incorporate alkali   L.E. cells
  reserve)
Bilirubin from Rhesus babies   Serum iron and total
Bleeding   iron binding capacity
Blood count   Sternal marrow
Blood culture   puncture (laboratory
Blood sugar (glucose)   technician present)
                               Synacthen stimulation
                               test

Some blood tests are now carried out by the use of re-agent strips for example:

Azostix: indicates (a raised) blood urea level.
Dextrostix: a semi quantitative method for estimating blood sugar (glucose) levels. These tests are time saving, but it is essential that each detail of the instructions is followed and the timing must be critical, using a watch with a seconds hand accurately or the results may prove unreliable.

Blood Counts

Blood counts may be made by drawing blood directly from a finger prick into special pipettes which the operator brings to the bedside. More commonly, how-ever, venous blood is collected in a sequestrene tube and two thin blood smears prepared, for the differential count in the laboratory. This second method is more convenient, as several other examinations can be made from the same specimen if they are required. Usually 2 to 3 ml are collected. (For Normal Values see p. 183.)

Erythrocyte Sedimentation Rate

The sedimentation rate measures the distance which the

red cells fall in one hour when a column of blood is allowed to stand vertically in a glass tube of fine uniform bore. Several different methods are used, and the normal values vary with each method. It is not a diagnostic test, as most infections cause an increase in the rate, but it is very useful in following the course of a disease— e.g. in rheumatic fever and tuberculosis. The greater the activity of the disease the higher is the sedimentation rate.

Wintrobe's method is the one most used. 3 ml of blood are placed in a tube containing ammonium and potassium oxalate, and well mixed. A special Wintrobe sedimentation rate tube is then filled and allowed to stand vertically undisturbed for 1 hour, and then the height of the column of clear plasma above the sediment of red cells is measured.

Another method is the Westergren method, where 0·4 ml of a 3% sodium citrate solution is used for the anticoagulant and a different size tube is used. (For Normal Values see p. 183.)

Bleeding time is the duration of bleeding after puncturing the ear lobe, which is usually 1 to 4 minutes. It may, however, be prolonged in patients with thrombocytopenia. *Clotting or coagulation time* is the period taken for one drop of blood to coagulate, which is usually 4½ minutes. Other more complex clotting functions can be measured by means of special tests. One of these is used to estimate prothrombin concentration for the control of anti-coagulant treatments.

Bone Marrow Specimens

Samples of bone marrow may be required in cases of pernicious anaemia and leukaemia. These are obtained by puncturing the manubrium sterni or the iliac crest with a sternal puncture needle and aspirating the bone marrow. (The patient is usually given a sedative—e.g. Seconal 200 mg or Physeptone 10 mg, 45 to 60 minutes before the procedure is carried out.) A member of the laboratory staff usually prepares the smears.

Plasma Proteins

Disturbances of the plasma proteins occur in many conditions. Abnormally low levels of serum albumin may give rise to oedema and may be the result of liver diseases, loss of albumin in the urine in the nephrotic syndrome, or a diet deficient in proteins.

Serum protein levels are often low in patients with chronic infections or extensive burns. Raised or abnormal globulins are found in patients with multiple myelomas.

Plasma Cortisol Estimations (11-hydroxy corticosteroids). This is usually performed in preference to urinary ketosteroids; a specific steroid hormone can then be estimated rather than a complex mixture of steroids and metabolites. This is a test of adrenal cortical function in Addison's and Simmonds' disease. Levels are usually highest in the morning so that a suitable time for taking blood which is collected into a special 10 ml tube, would be between 8.0 a.m. and 9 a.m.

Plasma Electrolytes. (See p. 30.)

Serous Fluids

Pleural effusions, pericardial effusions and ascitic fluid are formed in a number of conditions.

Microscopic, bacteriological and chemical investigations of these fluids are used to determine the nature of the underlying disorder.

Cell content. In transudates only a small number of cells is present. In pyogenic infections pus cells are present in large numbers, while in tuberculous infection there is a high percentage of lymphocytes. Red blood cells are often present in malignant disease.

Bacteriological investigations. In infective conditions culture for pyogenic organisms or the *Mycobacterium tuberculosis* may reveal the organism responsible for the infection. For the detection of tuberculous infection the fluid may be injected into guinea-pigs.

Chemical examinations. The protein content is increased in infective conditions, but may also be raised to a lesser extent in transudates.

Pleural Biopsy

Biopsy of the parietal pleura may be needed in order to determine whether a pleural effusion is tuberculous or malignant in origin.

The biopsy needle is usually inserted into the posterior chest wall; the exact site is decided after physical and radiological examination. The patient should sit well forward in the bed with his arms resting on a pillow placed on a bed table in front of him. A labelled bottle containing formalin is required for the specimen.

Bacteriological Examinations

In many conditions specimens are required for bacteriological examination in order to identify the micro-organisms responsible, for example, throat, nose and wound swabs, sputum, stools, pleural and cerebrospinal fluid.

Table of Sensitivity of
Common Micro-organisms to Antibiotics

Note: This table is basically correct but the range of antibiotics is now so wide that it is impracticable to include all. Micro-organism	Penicillin	Streptomycin	Tetracycline group	Chloramphenicol	Erythromycin	Sulphonamide
Streptococcus haemolyticus	++	V	+	+	+	+
Streptococcus viridans	V	V	+	+	+	V
Staphylococcus pyogenes	V	V	V	V	+	+
Pneumococcus	++	V	+	+	+	+
Clostridium group (tetanus, gas gangrene)	++	O	+	+	+	+
Corynebacterium diphtheriae	+	O	+	+	+	O
Neisseria gonorrhoeae	++	+	+	+	+	+
Meningococcus	+	O	+	+	+	++
Haemophilus influenzae	O	++	+	+	+	+
Haemophilus pertussis (whooping cough)	O	++	+	+	+	+
Escherichia coli (urinary infections)	O	+	+	+	O	++
Salmonella typhi (typhoid fever)	O	O	V	++	O	FO
Salmonella paratyphi (paratyphoid fever)	O	O	V	++	O	O
Shigella group (bacillary dysentery)	O	+	++	++	O	+
Treponema pallidum (syphilis)	++	O	+	+	O	O
*Mycobacterium tuberculosis**	O	++	O	O	O	O
Rickettsia group (typhus fever)	O	O	++	++	+	O

++ = very sensitive.   + = sensitive.   V = variable.   O = insensitive

* Also sensitive to Para-aminosalicylic Acid (PAS) and Isoniazid.

These specimens must be collected under strict aseptic conditions and in sterile containers. An exception to this is the collection of a specimen of faeces, while the entire stool may be sent to the laboratory labelled in the bed-pan in which it is passed, or a small quantity of the material (particularly mucus, pus and blood if present) is sent to the laboratory in a screw-capped container. When taking swabs for bacteriological examination care must be taken to ensure that no antiseptic is applied to the surface for several hours prior to swabbing. If the patient is under treatment by any chemotherapeutic agent at the time this should be stated.

All specimens will be examined by direct smear and by culture; information can also be obtained with regard to the sensitivity of organisms to the various antibiotics. (See Table on p. 156.)

Digestive System

Tests of Gastric Function

These tests are designed to estimate the hydrochloric acid content of the gastric juice and the amount and content of the gastric residuum ('resting juice') after a period of fasting. The tests vary from one hospital to another and even according to the doctor who orders them. Some examples are given below:

Diagnex test (also known as the 'tubeless' test). No preparations containing aluminium, calcium, iron or magnesium must be given during the 24 hours prior to the test. The patient should fast for 12 hours before the commencement of the test and should have nothing but the test substances and water by mouth until the test is complete.

1. At the specified time (e.g. 6 a.m.) the patient is asked to empty his bladder and this urine is discarded.

2. He is given 2 capsules containing caffeine sodium benzoate 250 mg with a glass of water. This preparation is a gastric stimulant.

3. If an injection of histamine has been ordered it is given at 6.45 a.m.

4. At 7 a.m. the patient again empties his bladder, the entire amount passed is saved and sent to the laboratory in a container labelled 'control urine'.

5. Immediately after emptying his bladder the patient is given the 'Diagnex' (Azure A Resin) blue granules suspended in about 60 ml (2 fluid ounces) of water. The granules do not dissolve and thus the patient must be instructed not to chew them but to swallow them whole. A further 60 ml of water is given to ensure that no granules are left in the glass.

6. Two hours later, 9 a.m., the patient empties his bladder and all the urine passed is saved and sent to the laboratory in a container labelled 'test urine'.

If the gastric juice contains hydrochloric acid an exchange of hydrogen ions can be effected with the azure A resin in the test substance. Azure A resin is then absorbed and excreted in the urine.

The test cannot be repeated until at least a week has elapsed and therefore the nurse should be sure that she understands the instructions and carries them out accurately.

The patient may continue to pass blue or greenish-blue urine for some days after the test.

Fractional test meal. This type of test is now less commonly used. It is usually carried out in the early morning and the patient should be given nothing by mouth for at least 8 hours.

A series of specimen bottles, or test tubes, is needed, one is labelled 'resting juice' and the remainder are numbered 1 to 12.

1. A Ryle's or other intragastric tube is passed and the 'resting juice' aspirated. A sample is placed in the labelled test tube.

2. If alcohol is used for the test meal, 200 ml of 5% or 50 ml 7% alcohol is injected down the intragastric tube. Gruel (made by boiling 60 g (2 oz) of fine oatmeal with one litre of water until the volume is reduced to half a litre (500 ml)) is sometimes used, in which case this is given to the patient to drink with the intragastric tube left in position. Histamine or soluble insulin may be prescribed by the doctor as gastric stimulants. When insulin is used blood sugar estimations are made before administration and 20 minutes and 40 minutes afterwards.

3. A sample (about 5 ml) of gastric content is aspirated every 15 minutes and put in the appropriate test tube beginning with No. 1.

Residual contents are finally aspirated and the series of test tubes in a labelled rack is sent to the laboratory. The procedure usually takes 2 or 3 hours. The results of the test will include an analysis of the 'resting juice' and the amount of free hydrochloric acid in the successive specimens aspirated.

Histamine may produce unpleasant symptoms such as generalized flushing and throbbing in the head as a result of its vasodilator action. These symptoms can be prevented by giving one of the anti-histamine drugs, e.g. promethazine hydrochloride (Phenergan). A glucose drink should be available for a patient showing severe symptoms of hypoglycaemia.

Overnight Suction for Gastric Analysis

Augmented histamine test meal

The patient is starved from 6 p.m.

At 9 p.m.	A Ryle's tube is passed and attached to a suction machine. Aspiration of gastric content continues throughout the night.
At 9 a.m.	The tube is spigoted for 1 hour.
At 10 a.m.	The fluid aspirated is labelled 'Resting juice'. Suction then continues until 11 a.m. this aspirated fluid is labelled 'Specimen 1'.
At 10.30 a.m.	A 100 mg of Anthisan is given intramuscularly.
At 11.5 a.m.	Histamine 0·04 mg per kg body weight is given intramuscularly. Suction continues with 3 more specimens of gastric juice collected at $\frac{1}{2}$-hourly intervals for $1\frac{1}{2}$ hours. Any residual contents are then collected and labelled and all the specimens sent to the laboratory.

Analysis of Faeces for Blood (Occult Blood)

Bleeding from peptic ulcer or a new growth is not detectable by the naked eye examination of the stool if the blood lost is very small in amount and mixed with the intestinal contents.

Tests of Intestinal and Pancreatic Function

The absorption of various food materials, especially fats, may be impaired in diseases of the small intestine or of the pancreas, and several tests are in use to measure the efficiency of intestinal absorption.

Analysis of Faeces for Fat

Specimens of faeces must be inspected before submitting them for quantitative analysis. The highly fluid stools obtained by means of purgatives and enemas are useless. No aperients and particularly no oily preparations such as liquid paraffin should be used for several days before a specimen is sent for fat estimation and barium should have been expelled following a Barium Meal. On occasions when the whole stool cannot conveniently be forwarded, the material available must be mixed to a uniform consistency and a 30 g (1 oz) sample sent in an airtight container.

On a normal diet the total daily output of fat should be less than 7 g. In some circumstances estimation of the faecal fat on a free diet may not provide a sufficiently accurate result and in this event a fat balance test will be necessary.

Fat Balance Test

The patient is given a standard diet, containing 50 g fat per day, during the test and for at least 48 hours prior to its commencement. It is essential that all the food be ingested or any rejects returned to the diet kitchen.

1st day of test. The patient is given 2 capsules containing carmine before breakfast.

The stools are examined as passed and when they are coloured by carmine the whole stool is saved and sent to the laboratory. All subsequent stools are saved for six days.

6th day of test. The patient is given 60 g (2 oz) of charcoal powder mixed with water. All stools passed are saved until charcoal appears in the faeces.

A convenient method of collecting the stools is into a sheet of cellophane placed in the bed-pan and large enough to hang down covering the rim. The edges of the sheet are brought together and the whole stool in the cellophane is deposited in a labelled, waterproof container.

Normally, 91–99% of the ingested fat is absorbed.

NOTE. Liquid paraffin and oily drugs must not be given during the test, or for at least 3 days prior to its commencement.

Other Malabsorption Tests

The absorption of substances other than fat may also be impaired. Carbohydrate absorption is measured by a xylose tolerance test. The patient should fast for 12 hours before the test. He then takes 5·0 g of this substance, which is a relatively inert carbohydrate, in a drink of fruit juice, having first emptied the bladder. All the urine passed in the following 5 hours is collected and sent to the laboratory. During this time, the patient is encouraged to drink water but does not eat. The 5-hour specimen of urine should contain at least 1·2 g of xylose, but if uptake of this substance from the gut is impaired, less than this amount will be present in the urine.

A number of vitamins are absorbed from the bowel, and the body may become deficient in them in states of abnormal intestinal function. If vitamin K is absorbed poorly the prothrombin concentration in the plasma falls and a bleeding tendency may develop. Poor absorption of vitamin B^{12}, deficiency of which leads to pernicious anaemia, is tested by administering a very small dose of radioactive vitamin B^{12} and measuring its excretion in the urine (*Schilling test*).

Intestinal Biopsy

The intestinal wall is abnormal in conditions such as coeliac disease or idiopathic steatorrhoea and a specimen may be obtained by means of an instrument known as the Crosby capsule. The capsule contains a cutting mechanism actuated through a long thin flexible tube. It is usually swallowed at about 10 p.m., the patient having fasted since 6 p.m. From the stomach it progresses about 5 cm (2″) per hour. The position is checked in the morning by X-ray and the biopsy taken from the appropriate site by applying suction to the tube.

Pancreatic Function

The internal secretion of the pancreas, insulin, is disturbed in diabetes mellitus, but is not usually affected by other diseases of the pancreas unless the organ has been extensively destroyed. This aspect of pancreatic function is considered under 'Carbohydrate Metabolism' on p. 175.

The external secretions of the pancreas may be tested either by estimating the amylase content of the blood or urine or by analysis of the duodenal contents for pancreatic enzymes and bicarbonates.

Urinary Amylase

A sample of the urine collected over several hours is desirable. When, however, it is a matter of urgency, as, for example, for the confirmation of a diagnosis of acute pancreatitis, examination of the first specimen obtained is permissible. If the urine has to be sent some distance to the laboratory it should be preserved with benzene.

The normal range of urinary diastase is from 6 to 30 units per ml. A value of 200 or more units in a case with acute abdominal signs is almost pathognomonic of acute pancreatitis. Intermediate values between 30 and 200, if found regularly, may be useful in directing attention to the possibility of pancreatic duct obstruction.

Duodenal Drainage

A more detailed examination of the pancreatic function may be carried out by examination of the duodenal juice obtained by duodenal drainage. A weighted duodenal tube is passed into the stomach and a specimen of gastric juice is withdrawn. The patient then lies on his right side to promote the passage of the tube into the duodenum. If necessary the position of the tube can be checked by X-ray. When the tube is in the duodenum the contents are aspirated and tested for sodium bicarbonate and the pancreatic enzymes, trypsin, amylase and lipase. Pancreatic secretion may be stimulated by a subcutaneous injection of Mecholyl or an intravenous injection of Secretin.

Liver Function

Tests of liver function are less satisfactory than function tests of some other organs because the liver has numerous functions, any single one of which may be deficient, whilst the others remain relatively intact. Also the liver has a large reserve and has to be very extensively damaged before any of the tests show an abnormal result. No test has yet been devised which tests the liver as a whole, but there are innumerable tests which depend on the different individual functions of the organ. The commonest of these tests are given below.

Bile Pigments

Failure of the liver to excrete bile pigments leads to the

accumulation of these in the blood and their excretion in the urine.

1. **Bilirubin.** The normal level of bilirubin in the blood serum varies from 0·2 to 0·75 mg per 100 ml. Increased serum bilirubin is found in liver damage, obstructive jaundice and haemolytic jaundice.

Bilirubin will be present in the urine in all cases of jaundice except haemolytic jaundice.

2. **Urobilinogen.** This pigment will be present in the urine in cases of incomplete obstructive jaundice, in diffuse liver damage, for example infective hepatitis and in haemolytic jaundice. In cases of complete obstructive jaundice urobilinogen is absent from the urine.

For urine tests for bile pigments see p. 147.

Serum Protein Tests

These tests are designed to show variations from the normal ability of the liver to synthesize serum proteins. They are not specific tests for liver damage since alterations in the serum proteins may be found in many other diseases.

In liver diseases the serum albumin level is low and the serum globulin is raised. The abnormal composition of the serum proteins is also reflected in the so-called 'empirical liver function tests', for example the Thymol Turbidity test. These become positive when liver function is impaired—e.g. in cirrhosis of the liver and infective hepatitis.

Bromsulphthalein Test

This test measures the ability of the liver to excrete a dye, bromsulphthalein.

The patient should have a fat-free breakfast and no food thereafter until the test is completed.

10.00 a.m. 5 mg per kilogram of body weight of 5%
            bromsulphthalein is injected intravenously
            very slowly over a period of 3 minutes. The
            ampoule must be warmed if any crystals are
            visible.

10.45 a.m. 10 ml of clotted blood is collected from
            another vein, special care being taken to
            avoid haemolysis.

Interpretation of the test. After 45 minutes the serum
should show that less than 7% of the injected dose is
still retained.

Prothrombin Concentration Test

Prothrombin is formed in the liver from vitamin K
absorbed from the intestine. A low prothrombin may be
due to liver damage, or to the non-absorption of vitamin K resulting from biliary obstruction. If the prothrombin concentration is low, the test may be repeated
after an injection of vitamin K, and if it then returns to
normal it is suggestive of biliary obstruction. The prothrombin level must also be estimated regularly in
patients having anticoagulant therapy.

Liver Biopsy

Prior to carrying out this investigation the patient's
blood group is ascertained, his blood is cross-matched,
the haemoglobin and prothrombin content, the bleeding time and the clotting time are estimated. (The biopsy
is not usually proceeded with if the prothrombin content
is found to be below 70% of the normal.)

  The patient lies on his back well over to the right side
of the bed, a pillow is placed under his left side to tilt
the trunk slightly to the right.

Bleeding into the peritoneal cavity may occur following liver biopsy and therefore the patient must be under close observation, an hourly pulse chart should be kept for at least 12 hours following this procedure.

Renal Function

Ordinary chemical and microscopic examination of the urine, although valuable, gives only limited information as to the condition of the kidneys. Albuminuria, for example, may be met with apart from nephritic condition, and in nephritis it is not always possible to form an opinion merely from simple chemical examination of the urine, whether the kidneys are functioning properly. In spite of a large excretion of urea, uric acid, creatinine and other end products of nitrogenous metabolism, the level of these substances in the blood may be much above normal; in such cases it is only by reason of this increased 'head' that the kidneys are able to excrete their daily quota of waste substances. Tests have, therefore, been devised with the object either of directly estimating renal efficiency or of investigating the severity and following the progress of events in a nephritic lesion.

Blood Urea Estimation

2·5 ml of blood is collected from a vein into a sequestrene tube to prevent coagulation.

With smaller quantities of blood reasonably satisfactory results can be obtained when the urea content is high, but the results in borderline cases cannot be regarded as sufficiently accurate.

If this test is done in conjunction with a urea concentration test the blood sample must be taken before the draught is given.

The normal range of variation of blood urea is from 20 to 40 mg per 100 ml. Some authorities allow up to 60 mg in elderly patients.

Low values occur in normal pregnancy and in acute yellow atrophy, but may also be produced by protein deprivation and flushing out the system with water as in diabetes insipidus or diuresis produced by high fluid intake.

High values of 100 mg per 100 ml or more nearly always indicate serious renal impairment, but moderate increases can occur without renal involvement in dehydration, circulatory failure and high protein intake. In cases with some degree of renal damage wide fluctuations in blood urea content can be produced by variations in protein and water intake, so that the fall which occurs when a nephritic patient is placed on a low protein liquid diet is not necessarily an indication of fundamental improvement.

Urea Concentration Test (Maclean)

The intake of fluids should be restricted as much as possible from the afternoon preceding the test. No breakfast is allowed.

In the morning, blood is collected for urea estimation. (See previous test.)

The patient empties the bladder and a sample of this urine is placed in a bottle labelled '1'.

He is now given 15 g ($\frac{1}{2}$ oz) of urea dissolved in about 60 ml (2 oz) water. (A smaller dose for children in proportion to age.)

At intervals of 1 hour from taking the urea draught the patient empties the bladder. Three specimens marked ('2', '3' and '4') are obtained in this way and sent in labelled containers.

The blood must be collected *before* the urea draught is given.

Specimens sent from a distance should be preserved by adding a few drops of benzene.

Some authorities prefer to discard the urine passed during the first hour after the draught and consider only the results for the second, third and fourth hours.

A figure of 2% or over in one or more of the hour specimens is regarded as evidence of satisfactory renal function. Diuresis sometimes prevents this concentration being reached and if the volume exceeds 120 ml (4 oz) a concentration of urea below 2% does not necessarily indicate poor function. The restriction of fluids is designed to prevent diuresis, and ignoring the first hour specimen, in which diuresis is often most marked, also aims at overcoming this difficulty.

Urea Clearance Test

Two methods are used, one without and one with urea, the aim of the latter being to impose a load on the kidneys to provoke maximum efficiency. The need for this is denied by some authorities. In either case the test should be done before breakfast is taken. The details of these tests may vary in different hospitals. Two methods are given below:

First method (without urea). The patient empties the bladder completely at 8 a.m. Discard the urine.

At 9 a.m. the patient empties the bladder completely. Place the *whole* specimen directly into a container without measurement. Mark the bottle 'A'.

A specimen of blood is collected immediately for urea estimation.

At 10 a.m. the patient again empties the bladder

completely. Place the *whole* specimen directly without measurement into a container. Mark the bottle 'B'.

Second method (with urea). The patient empties the bladder at 8 a.m. Discard the urine. Give immediately a draught containing 15 g of urea. (A smaller dose for children according to age.)

At 9 a.m. the patient empties the bladder completely. Discard this urine.

At 9.45 a.m. a specimen of blood is collected for urea estimation.

At 10 a.m. the patient empties the bladder completely. Place the *whole* specimen directly without measurement into a clean bottle.

Greater sensitivity is claimed for this test, but, as might be expected, this increased sensitivity will not be realized in practice unless close attention is given to detail.

The patient must be asked to make special efforts to empty the bladder completely at the times specified.

These times must be noted accurately—e.g. to the nearest minute—and recorded on the slip to accompany the specimens for the information of the laboratory. The intervals need not be precisely 1 hour if this request is complied with.

The urine must be poured as completely as possible into the specimen bottles, for the total amount is accurately measured in the laboratory and any loss of urine will produce a low result.

The specimens of urine may be preserved if necessary by the addition of three or four drops of benzene.

In the case of children and unusually small or large adults the height and weight may also be required by the laboratory for the calculation of the result.

Analysis of the specimens submitted gives figures from which the efficiency of the kidneys is calculated, the result being in terms of the percentage of average normal renal function. The common range in normal health is from 75 to 120%. Cases of acute nephritis have been studied by means of this test. The patients show a marked fall in the urea clearance, sometimes as low as 10% during the early weeks of the acute stage and, while fatal cases show a continued fall, a rise in the clearance value is accompanied by clinical improvement. The active chronic phase of the disease is indicated by a progressively diminishing urea clearance, uraemia and death being imminent when values below 10% are obtained. The renal failure found in some cases of hypertension is also associated with a falling urea clearance test, while in nephrosis no impairment of function is found.

With this, as with all other tests of kidney function, sight must not be lost of the fact that the result indicates the state of affairs on the day of the test only and that the condition may be changing extremely rapidly.

Urine Concentration Test

No fluids are allowed from 4 p.m. on the preceding day until 8 a.m. on the morning of the test. The patient empties his bladder at 8, 9 and 10 a.m. and the volume and specific gravity of each specimen is measured. The specific gravity of at least one specimen should exceed 1025 if renal function is normal. This test should not be done if the blood urea is raised.

Renal Biopsy

Prior to this procedure an X-ray examination is carried out in order to obtain information about the size and position of the kidneys; the patient's blood group is ascertained, his blood is cross-matched and the haemoglobin content estimated.

The patient lies in the prone position with a sandbag under the abdomen to fix the kidney against the dorsal surface of the body.

The site of the biopsy is usually the lower pole of the right kidney and its position is ascertained by a fine exploring needle inserted after the injection of a local anaesthetic.

Haematuria is not uncommon after renal biopsy: the appearance of blood in the urine, even if slight in amount, should be reported at once. An hourly pulse chart should be kept for at least 12 hours.

Ascorbic acid saturation test. This is carried out on patients with ascorbic acid deficiency, who may take more than seven days to reach saturation. It is repeated daily until the patient excretes more than 30 mg of ascorbic acid in the 2-hour specimen.

8 a.m.   The patient empties the bladder and is given 700 mg ascorbic acid by mouth.

12 noon   The patient empties the bladder and the specimen is discarded.

2 p.m.   The patient empties the bladder and all the urine passed is collected into a special container (which contains 50 ml of glacial acetic acid). The ascorbic acid content must be estimated within one hour.

Figlu test. This is carried out to detect folic acid deficiency. Histidine monohydrochloride 15 g is given by mouth after overnight fasting and food is withheld until one hour after administration of the dose. As the

Histadine is only slightly soluble it is administered by mixing it with water until all has been taken. Three hours after taking the dose, the patient voids urine and this is discarded. All urine passed over the next five hours (i.e. three to eight hours after the histadine dose) is collected into a special container which contains N/10 hydrochloric acid and a few crystals of thymol.

Catechol amines. This test is undertaken to estimate the amines, adrenaline and noradrenaline in the urine in suspected cases of phaeochromocytoma, a tumour of the adrenal medulla. A 24-hour specimen of urine is collected into a special container in which there is dilute acid.

17-Ketosteroids (oxosteroids) and 17-Ketogenic steroids (oxogenic steroids). These are tests of adrenal cortical dysfunction which are carried out on a 24-hour specimen of urine.

Bence-Jones protein. This test is used in the diseases of multiple myeloma and secondary carcinoma of bone. A special type of protein appears in the urine when it is heated to 50 °C and redissolves as boiling point is reached. Since albumin is often present in addition, this redissolving on boiling may be difficult to detect except by using special laboratory methods.

Slide pregnancy test. Early morning urine is best for this test as it is more concentrated. It should be collected into a sterile bottle and sent to the laboratory without delay. Some laboratories accept a bottle which has previously been boiled and is free from detergent. The test is not normally positive until after 41 days from the date of the last menstrual period.

Cerebrospinal Fluid

For complete routine examination 5–10 ml of cerebro-spinal fluid should be sent to the laboratory.

The following points should be borne in mind in col-lecting these specimens:

contamination with blood detracts from the value of the report in proportion to the amount present;

dilution of the fluid with water, saline, spirit and other fluids must be rigidly avoided;

bacterial contamination invalidates some of the tests such as sugar content and the colloidal gold test.

Cell count. In normal fluid there are usually a few white cells (lymphocytes) present, 0 to 5 per cubic millimetre. Pus cells are found in pyogenic infections, and lympho-cytes are increased in tuberculous meningitis, syphilitic infections, and poliomyelitis. Red blood cells will be found in cases of subarachnoid haemorrhage and in cerebral haemorrhage if blood has leaked into the ventricles.

Protein. This is increased in infective conditions, syphil-itic lesions and spinal block.

Glucose. The normal range is from 50 to 85 mg per cent. It is usually low or absent in infective and tuberculous meningitis. Slightly raised values are said to occur in encephalitis lethargica; in subjects with raised blood sugar the spinal fluid sugar is also raised.

Sodium chlorate. The normal range is 720 to 750 mg per 100 ml. Values tend to be reduced in acute menin-gitis and in the late stages of tuberculous meningitis. In syphilitic conditions normal values are the rule.

Lange's colloidal gold reaction. No precipitation of gold occurs with normal fluid in any dilution. The degree of precipitation is reported numerically, 0 indicating no and 5 complete precipitation. In general paralysis of the insane the gold is precipitated by the lower dilutions in a standard series, the report being of the type 55554210000 (paretic curve), while meningitic fluids usually show the greatest change in the higher dilutions, the report reading 00002355555.

Carbohydrate Metabolism

The following tests are used to detect disturbances of carbohydrate metabolism, in particular in diabetes.

Estimation of Blood Sugar

This test should be done in the morning before food has been taken.

If the patient is unable to visit the laboratory, $\frac{1}{2}$ ml of blood may be sent in a small tube (supplied on request) containing a special preservative mixture. The tube must be shaken thoroughly to mix the blood with the preservative.

NOTE: Blood without this preservative powder (5 parts sodium fluoride, 1 part powdered thymol) is useless for this test, as the sugar content begins to diminish within an hour.

Where repeated observations are to be made, as during adjustment of diet and insulin dosage, specimens must always be taken in the same relation to the previous meal and insulin, in order that the results may be comparable. This may be 3 hours after the meal, or in the morning before breakfast.

The great majority of normal fasting blood-sugar values lie between 80 to 120 mg per 100 ml. It has been found, almost without exception, that values of 130 mg per ml or more are found only in those cases which give a 'diabetic curve' in the glucose tolerance test. Some cases of hyperthyroidism, or patients on therapeutic thyroid dosage, also give high results, whilst apprehension on appearing at the laboratory for the first time is occasionally responsible. Very low values are found after an excessive dose of insulin, following severe exercise, or in the rare condition of hyper-insulinism.

Glucose Tolerance Test

The way in which an individual is able to deal with a standard quantity of sugar affords valuable information as to the presence, or otherwise, of a diabetic tendency. It is desirable that the test should be done in the morning before food has been taken. Extremes of high or low carbohydrate diet should be avoided for at least one day before the test. Nervous tension and rush before and during the test should be discouraged and smoking must be forbidden.

The patient may be sent to the laboratory by appointment for the test or, where this is not practicable, the following procedure must be adopted:

The patient empties the bladder. A sample of this urine is placed in a bottle marked 'A'.

A 0·5 ml sample of blood is collected in a special blood-sugar tube. (See previous section.)

50 g of glucose is given, dissolved in 100 ml of water (about 4 oz). (For children a smaller dose according to age.)

At ½-hour intervals thereafter, five more samples of blood are collected.

The patient empties the bladder one hour and two hours after the administration of glucose. These specimens are placed in bottles labelled 'B' and 'C'.

When the urine specimens are sent from a distance to the laboratory for testing they should be preserved with a few drops of benzene.

A normal individual should show a fasting sugar between 80 and 120 mg per 100 ml, a definite rise during the first hour and a return to fasting limits within 2 hours. The maximum reading should not exceed 180 mg per 100 ml and no sugar should be found in the specimens of urine.

Diabetes mellitus. The initial blood-sugar level may be normal or raised, the rise after the administration of glucose continues about 180 mg per 100 ml and the blood sugar remains above the fasting range for more than 2 hours.

In the majority of diabetic patients, the first specimen of urine 'A' contains no sugar, this appears in the later specimens ('B' and 'C').

Renal glycosuria. In this condition the initial blood sugar is normal or subnormal, and does not rise above 180 mg per 100 ml and the return to fasting limits is not delayed, being often more rapid than usual; sugar is not present in the first specimen of urine except in unusual cases with very low renal threshold, but is invariably present in the second specimen. It is almost universally agreed that this fairly common condition is of no pathological significance. One of the values of the glucose tolerance test lies in recognizing these cases and saving them the rigours of diabetic treatment.

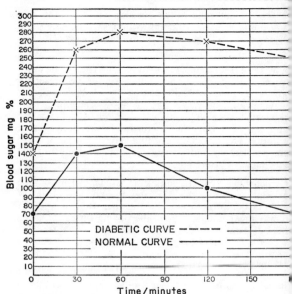

BLOOD-SUGAR CURVES

Hyperthyroidism and pituitary disturbances. Abnormal blood-sugar curves are sometimes found in these conditions.

Glycosuria of pregnancy. In a fair percentage of normal pregnancies glycosuria is found while the blood sugar remains normal.

In the various uncommon conditions in which reducing substances other than glucose are present in the urine, for example pentose, the tolerance test usually gives a normal result.

Calcium Metabolism

The commoner causes of disturbed calcium metabolism are diseases of the parathyroid glands, failure of absorption of calcium due to steatorrhoea, vitamin D deficiency and chronic renal disease.

In the condition of hyperparathyroidism due to tumours of the parathyroid glands, calcium is lost from the bones leading to osteomalacia and a raised serum calcium level. In these cases the blood phosphorus is low and the alkaline phosphatase level in the blood is raised. In tetany due to absence of the parathyroid hormone blood calcium is low.

In steatorrhoea there is a failure of absorption of calcium from the gut which gives rise to low blood calcium and osteomalacia.

The administration of vitamin D aids calcium absorption, but excessive dosage can cause a raised level of the blood calcium.

Laboratory tests used in disordered calcium metabolism include estimation of the blood calcium, the blood phosphorus, the blood alkaline phosphatase, and the Calcium balance. This latter test involves a somewhat complicated routine as detailed in the following instructions.

Calcium Balance Routine

The patient is on a weighed and analysed diet. The tray is delivered to the patient and collected by the dietician, who weighs any rejects. The diet is the same throughout the test. The whole of it must be eaten. Nothing extra is allowed.

The water is distilled for drinking. As much as the patient likes may be given. All food is cooked in distilled water in utensils kept solely for this purpose. No toothpaste may be used, distilled water mouthwashes are substituted.

The patient is on this routine for 6 days before collections are begun. This is the equilibrium period during which time small alterations may be made in the diet to suit the patient's taste.

At 6 a.m. on the first day of the specimen collection, the patient empties the bladder. This urine is rejected. All subsequent specimens are collected in 24-hourly bottles, the last specimen of each 24 hours being obtained at 6 a.m. after which a new bottle is begun. Each bottle contains 10 ml toluol to preserve the urine.

The evening before the start of the collections a carmine cachet is given to colour the faeces. This is given the evening before the end of each balance period. Following this all stools are saved in individual containers and the balance periods are considered to be from the end of the marked (red) stool to the end of the second marked stool.

Urine and faeces must be collected separately. The bed-pan is rinsed in distilled water before being used by the patient. After use it is cleaned in the normal way and rinsed in distilled water again. All faeces passed must be saved. The bed-pan is lined with cellophane to facilitate this.

No drugs to be given unless charted. All drugs given must be analysed. The advisability of giving such drugs should be checked before administration.

This routine may be modified to allow balance tests of other substances to be carried out.

Serum Enzymes

A vast number of enzymes is involved in cellular processes, but only very small amounts are found in the blood. When cells, particularly those in muscle and liver, are damaged, however, the concentration of certain enzymes in the blood rises and estimation of the relevant enzyme helps to establish the existence or amount of cellular damage. Those most commonly estimated are the aspartate transaminase (glutamic oxaloacetic transaminase or S.G.O.T.), which is increased especially after myocardial infection and in hepatitis, and the aline transaminase (glutamic pyruvic transaminase or S.G.P.T.), which is increased especially in various forms of liver cell damage.

Phosphatase

Two forms of phosphatase enzyme are present in blood serum, the alkaline and the acid. The former is increased in bone diseases, such as hyperparathyroidism, bone tumours and Paget's disease; the latter is frequently increased in carcinoma of the prostate gland with secondary deposits. The laboratory should be told which form is required when sending the specimen.

Either form of phosphatase can be determined on the serum obtained from 5 to 6 ml of blood. The normal ranges vary with the method used for determination, and information will be given by the laboratory.

Tests of Thyroid Gland Function

Radioactive Iodine

A measured tracer dose of radioactive iodine (I^{131}) is given orally or occasionally intravenously, and the amount of 'take up' or concentration of the radioactive material by the thyroid gland is recorded by a Geiger counter sited over the thyroid area, two hours later. A patient with myxoedema is asked to return 24 hours after the administration of the radioactive iodine, as the 'take up' is much slower. The average normal P.B.I. is 4 to 7·5 micrograms per 100 ml.

The results of the test may be invalidated if the patient is given radiological contrast media, food containing iodine, thyroid preparations, perchlorates or thiocyanates or radioactive isotopes. Some of these preparations may affect the result of the test even if a considerable time elapses between their discontinuation and the test, as for example Lugol's iodine and contrast media; it is therefore advisable to have an interval of 4 weeks if at all possible before carrying out the test.

The patient should be given the following instructions:

1. No food containing iodine, such as onions, watercress, fish, should be eaten for at least 2 days before coming for this test.

2. Iodized throat tablets, cough linctus and any proprietary food said to have a high iodine content should also be avoided. If these have been taken during the past month, will you please inform the department at the time of making the appointment.

3. A light breakfast may be taken on the morning of the test.

Thyroglobulin Antibody (T.A.) Test

Thyroglobulin Antibody in the serum is associated with certain forms of hypothyroidism: primary myxoedema and Hashimoto's disease. The test is positive in these conditions and negative in cancer. 2 ml of clotted blood is sufficient.

23. Normal Values and Blood Chemistry

Normal Values

Blood

Red Cells

4·5–6 million per cu mm (men)
4·3–5·5 ,, ,, ,, (women)

Haemoglobin in g per 100 ml

15–16 (men)
13–15 (women)

Sedimentation Rate

Westergren, 3–5 mm (men); 4–7 mm (women) in 1 hr
Wintrobe, 0–9 mm (men); 0–20 mm (women) in 1 hr

White Cells. 5,000–10,000 per cu mm

Neutrophils	40–60%
Lymphocytes	20–40
Monocytes	4–8
Eosinophils	1–3
Basophils	0–1

Platelets

200,000–500,000 per cu mm

Bleeding Time

1–4 minutes (Duke)
Less than 4 minutes (Ivy)

Clotting Time

  5–15 minutes (Lee and White)

Blood Chemistry

Calcium	..	..	9–10 mg per 100 ml
Chlorides	..	.. (total)	580–620 mg per 100 ml
			(100–106 mEq/Litre)
Cholesterol	..	..	150–240 mg per 100 ml
Glucose	..	..	80–120 mg per 100 ml
Phosphatase, alkaline	..		3–12 units per 100 ml
			(King-Armstrong)
			2·0–4·5 units per 100 ml
			(Bodansky)
Phosphatase, acid	..		1–3 units per 100 ml
Phosphorus	..	..	3–4·5 mg per 100 ml
Potassium	..	..	14–20 mg per 100 ml
			(3·5–5 mEq/Litre)
Protein	..	.. (total)	6–8 g per 100 ml
Albumin	..	..	4·5–5·5 g per 100 ml
Globulin	..	..	1·5–3·0 g per 100 ml
Fibrinogen	..	..	0·2–0·6 g per 100 ml
Sodium	..	..	310–340 mg per 100 ml
			(136–145 mEq/Litre)
Urea	..	.. ..	20–40 mg per 100 ml
Uric acid	..	.. ..	3–6 mg per 100 ml

Cerebrospinal Fluid (obtained by lumbar puncture)

Pressure	.. ..	80–180 mm of water
Volume (in adults)		120–140 ml
Cells	.. ..	0–5 per cu mm
Chlorides	.. ..	700–750 mg per 100 ml
Glucose	.. ..	50–85 ,, ,,
Protein	.. ..	10–45 ,, ,,

Urine

Volume 600–2,000 ml in 24 hours (average 1,200 ml).
Reaction variable, pH 4·7–8·0, usually slightly acid (pH 6·0).
Specific gravity 1003–1030.

Index

Baillière's Nursing Books

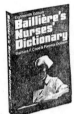

Baillière's Nurses' Dictionary

Cape & Dobson

The 18th edition of this famous dictionary has been completely reset and updated in a new format. It contains hundreds of new definitions, radically revised appendices and new illustrations — an informative, pocket-sized dictionary for student and trained nurse alike.

1974 • 18th edn. • Limp.

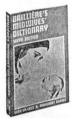

Baillière's Midwives' Dictionary

Da Cruz & Adams

The ideal pocket-sized dictionary for midwives and obstetric nurses. "A little mine of invaluable information...it really does contain the exact definition wanted in a hurry." *Midwives' Chronicle 1976 • 6th edn. • Limp.*

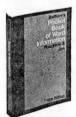

Baillière's Pocket Book of Ward Information

Fully revised and brought up-to-date, this book contains a multitude of useful information likely to be needed by nurses in their day to day work and of particular help to nurses in training.

1971 • 12th edn. • Limp.

The Nurses'
⊓⊓⊓ Aids Series

The Nurses' Aids Series is planned to meet the
needs of the student nurse during training, and
later in qualifying for another part of the
Register, by providing a set of textbooks
covering most of the subjects included in the
general part of the Register and certain
specialist subjects. The pupil nurse, too, will
find many of these books of particular value and
help in practical bedside training. The Series
conforms to three factors important to the
student:

1. All the authors are nurses who know exactly
what the student requires.
2. The books are frequently revised to ensure
that advances in knowledge reach the student
as soon as practicable.
3. The Aids are well printed and easy to read,
clearly illustrated, and modestly priced.

Anaesthesia & Recovery Room Techniques/Wachstein
1976 • 2nd edn.

Anatomy & Physiology for Nurses/Armstrong & Jackson
1972 • 8th edn.

Arithmetic in Nursing/Fream & Davies
1972 • 4th edn.

Ear, Nose & Throat Nursing/Marshall & Oxlade
1972 • 5th edn.

Geriatric Nursing/Storrs
1976 • 1st edn.

Medical Nursing/Chapman
1977 • 9th edn.

Microbiology for Nurses/Bocock & Parker
1972 • 4th edn.

For the Advanced Student

NURSES' AIDS SERIES SPECIAL INTEREST TEXTS

Special Interest Texts will enable the student nurse to study a particular subject in greater detail during training or after basic studies have been completed.

Gastroenterological Nursing/Gribble   1977 • 1st edn.

Neuromedical & Neurosurgical Nursing/Purchese   1977 • 1st edn.

Baillière's Medical Transparencies

* A visual reference library for lecturers and students.

* Of special interest to Nurses and Nurse Tutors are 'BMT 1', on the Anatomy of the Head, Neck and Limbs and 'BMT 2', on the Anatomy of the Thorax and Abdomen. Each set illustrates the major anatomical features of the regions with 21 and 18 slides in full colour. Other sets of interest to nurses specializing in these topics are **Paediatrics** 'BMT 17' and **Venereal Diseases** 'BMT 9' together with **Other Sexually Transmitted Diseases** 'BMT 19'. 24 slides in each set.

Quizzes and Questions for Nurses

Book A. Medical Nursing and Paediatric Nursing

Book B. Surgical Nursing and Geriatric Nursing

E. J. Hull and B. J. Isaacs

Two new books devised specially to help nurses in training to revise for examination purposes the subjects that they have been studying. The books are similar to the successful 'Do-It-Yourself' Revision series, but are set at a more elementary level. Each chapter is based on an examination question. The 'revision' part of each chapter consists of a quiz, with answers and explanations, covering the material to be revised.

1976 • Book A • 160pp. • 16 Illus. • Limp
Book B • 160pp. • 10 Illus. • Limp

Do-It-Yourself Revision For Nurses

Books 1, 2, 3, 4, 5 & 6

E. J. Hull and B. J. Isaacs

The six books of this series provide a comprehensive framework for revision of the GNC syllabus and developments made since to it. The student reviews a subject of choice, answers questions selected from recent State Final Examinations, and marks her replies against the model answers provided. 'Highly recommended to all student nurses as a planned guide to revision.' *Nursing Times.*

1970-1972 • Books 1-6 • 135pp average • illustrated

Standard Textbooks

Ward Administration & Teaching/Perry

"This is a book which has long been needed. Every trained nurse could learn something from it." *Nursing Mirror* 1968 • 1st edn.

Handbook of Practical Nursing/Crispin

This replaces the well-known textbook by Swire and is for the pupil and student nurse, written in a clear, easy-to-read style. 1976 • 1st edn.

Nursery Nursing — A A Handbook for Nursery Nurses/Meering & Stacey

"...a valuable reference book for all nurses interested in nursery work..." *The Lamp* 1971 • 5th edn.

Basic Nursing Care A Guide for Nursing Auxiliaries/Hutton

A practical, induction period, reference book for nursing auxiliaries in association with in-service training schemes and ward procedure manuals. 1974 • 1st edn.

Nursing in the Community/ Keywood

Provides a comprehensive account of the various problems peculiar to nursing outside the hospital, and describes the organization of a modern community nursing service. 1977 • 1st edn.

Books for the Psychiatric Nurse

Psychiatric Nursing/Altschul
Indispensable to students training for admission to the Register of Mental Nurses.
1977 • 5th edn. • 400pp. • Limp

Nursing the Psychiatric Patient/ Burr & Budge
For students in psychiatric training.
1976 • 3rd edn. • 320pp. • 15 illus. • Limp

Clinical Aspects of Dementia/ Pearce & Miller
Focuses on the treatable presenile dementias.
"Extremely useful" — Nursing Mirror
1973 • 160pp. • 12 plates, 15 illus.

Books for the Midwife

Mayes' Midwifery/Bailey
1976 • 9th edn. • 530pp. • 180 illus. • Limp

Obstetric & Gynaecological Nursing/Bailey
(Nurses' Aids Series)
1975 • 2nd edn. • 343pp. • 131 illus. • Limp

For Nurses Working in Intensive Care units

Patient Care: Cardiovascular Disorders/Ashworth & Rose
1973 • 309pp. • 110 illus.

Nurses' Guide to Cardiac Monitoring/Hubner
1975 • 2nd edn. • 66pp. • 37 illus. • Limp.

Cardiology/Julian
1973 • 2nd edn. • 341pp. • 112 illus. • Limp

Nursing Care of the Unconscious Patient/Mountjoy & Wythe
1970 • 104pp. • 11 illus. • Limp

A complete catalogue and current price lists are available on request direct from the publishers.

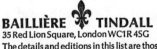

BAILLIÈRE TINDALL
35 Red Lion Square, London WC1R 4SG
The details and editions in this list are those
current at the time of going to press but are
liable to alteration without notice.

NOTES

NOTES

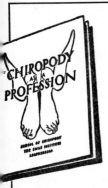